MW01231286

# Air Fryer Oven Cookbook

The best beginner's guide over 100 delicious recipes for homemade meals

Alice Frank

Table of Contents

# INTRODUCTION

Air fryers are the new and improved version of frying, healthier and faster than any way of cooking before it. Air fryers use just 30% oil to cook a variety of food, leaving the other 70% to be filled with flavor-producing moisture that would otherwise be lost in traditional deep-frying Directions. With an air fryer oven, you can easily make a whole meal without ever having to turn on the stove or oven. Utilizing an air fryer is a very simple and convenient process, but it does take some practice to learn the specifics. It requires little oil, little preparation time and produces a healthier meal. With the right air fryer oven, you can make all your favorite meals with ease in just minutes. There are different types of foods that can be cooked using an air fryer oven, including appetizers, snacks, pieces of bread, main courses and desserts. Whatever your cooking style, there is an air fryer oven out there for you. Cooking is a science and it takes time to learn how things work. Using an air fryer for the first time might be strange at first. It may yield some time getting used to, but once you get the hang of it you may find that it is just as easy and convenient as using a conventional oven or frying pan. Cooking times may vary. You can use a convection setting on an air fryer oven, and it is often recommended that this be done in order to cook more evenly and quickly. The surface temperature of food cooked in a convection mode is around 240°F, which is also high enough to burn the exterior of food quickly if not taken care of properly. Grilling outside is unhealthy and can create carcinogenic compounds. Using an indoor air fryer is the best way to cook without using oil. Ovens heat food above the temperature required to kill bacteria, while air fryers cook it at temperatures too low to produce those same harmful compounds. Cooking and serving food in air frying ovens reduce cooking time by many times over that of a conventional oven or stovetop. Using an air fryer to cook is much healthier than using oil and other fats. Using a standard convection oven, it takes about 3 tablespoons of oil to fry a chicken breast. The same chicken cooked in an air fryer takes about 5 tablespoons of oil - that's 25% less! Use just a couple of tsp. of olive oil and you'll be surprised how much flavor you can get out with so little. Cooking by means of an air fryer can be a healthier alternative to using other oils and fats. The latter are usually tropical in origin and contain saturated fats. To get the same amount of flavor out of last night's steak, you would need 10 times the amount of oil that comes from an air fryer in just a couple of teaspoons! In grilling using air fryer ovens, you can feed about 10 to 20 people with the air fryer which in comparison to the conventional ovens can only cook 3 to 6 people. The amount of time required for preparing and cooking a meal in an air fryer is significantly less than that of regular grills, and air fryers do not require much of any oil. Cooking times may differ reliant on the type and quantity of food being cooked, but usually, at temperatures amid 300°F and 400°F, the food will be ready in around 10 minutes. In baking using air fryer ovens, you can cook at 350°F for around 20 minutes and at 400°F for a little over half that time. In Roasting using an air fryer oven, you can do a large turkey around 18 pounds. The same in the conventional oven takes 35 to 50 minutes to get the same result, which is best if you want crispy skin.

# BREAKFAST AND BRUNCH

## 1. Egg Breakfast Ramekin

Preparation Time: 5 minutes Cooking Time: 8 minutes
Servings: 2

**Ingredients:**

2 tsp. unsalted butter (or coconut oil for dairy-free), for greasing
the ramekins  4 large eggs  2 tsp. chopped fresh thyme  ½ tsp.
fine sea salt  ¼ tsp. ground black pepper  2 tbsp. heavy cream
(or unsweetened, unflavored almond milk for dairy-free)  3
tbsp. finely grated Parmesan cheese (or Kite Hill brand chive
cream cheese style spread, softened, for dairy-free)  Fresh
thyme leaves, for garnish (optional)

**Directions:**

Preheat the air fryer to 400°F (205°C). Grease two 4-ounce
(113-g) ramekins with butter.  Crack 2 eggs into each ramekin
and divide the thyme, salt, and pepper between the ramekins.
Pour 1 tablespoon of the heavy cream into each ramekin.
Sprinkle each ramekin with 1½ tablespoons of the Parmesan
cheese.  Place the ramekins in the air fryer and cook for 8
minutes for soft-cooked yolks (longer if you desire a harder
yolk).  Garnish with a sprinkle of ground black pepper and
thyme leaves, if desired. Best served fresh.  Nutrition: Calories:
331 Fat: 29g Protein: 16g Carbs: 2g Net Carbs: 1g Fiber: 1g

## 2. Spaghetti Squash Patties

Preparation Time: 15 minutes Cooking Time: 8 minutes
Servings: 4

### Ingredients:

2 cups cooked spaghetti squash 2 tbsp. unsalted butter,
softened 1 large egg ¼ cup blanched finely ground almond
flour 2 stalks green onion, sliced ½ tsp. garlic powder 1 tsp.
dried parsley

### Directions:

Remove excess moisture from the squash using a cheesecloth or
kitchen towel. Mix all ingredients in a large bowl. Form into
four patties. Cut a piece of parchment to fit your air fryer
basket. Place each patty on the parchment and place it into the
air fryer basket. Adjust the temperature to 400°F (205°C) and
set the timer for 8 minutes. Flip the patties halfway through the
cooking time. Serve warm. Nutrition: Calories: 131 Fat: 10g
Protein: 4g Carbs: 7g Net Carbs: 5g Fiber: 2g

### 3. Breakfast Almond Cake

Preparation Time: 10 minutes Cooking Time: 7 minutes
Servings: 4

### Ingredients:

½ cup blanched finely ground almond flour ¼ cup powdered
erythritol ½ tsp. baking powder 2 tbsp. unsalted butter,
softened 1 large egg ½ tsp. unflavored gelatin ½ tsp. vanilla
extract ½ tsp. ground cinnamon

### Directions:

In a large bowl, mix almond flour, erythritol, and baking
powder. Add butter, egg, gelatin, vanilla, and cinnamon. Pour
into a 6-inch round baking pan. Place pan into the air fryer
basket. Adjust the temperature to 300°F (150°C) and set the
timer for 7 minutes. When the cake is completely cooked, a
toothpick will come out clean. Cut cake into four and Servings.
Nutrition: Calories: 153 Fat: 13g Protein: 5g Carbs: 13g Net
Carbs: 11g Fiber: 2g

## 4. Cheese and Bacon Quiche

Preparation Time: 5 minutes Cooking Time: 12 minutes
Servings: 2

### Ingredients:

3 large eggs  2 tbsp. heavy whipping cream  ¼ tsp. salt  4 slices
cooked sugar-free bacon, crumbled  ½ cup shredded mild
Cheddar cheese

### Directions:

In a large bowl, whisk eggs, cream, and salt together until
combined. Mix in bacon and Cheddar.  Pour mixture evenly into
two ungreased 4-inch ramekins. Place into air fryer basket.
Adjust the temperature to 320°F (160°C) and set the timer for
12 minutes. Quiche will be fluffy and set in the middle when
done.  Let quiche cool in ramekins 5 minutes. Serve warm.
Nutrition: Calories: 380 Fat: 28g Protein: 24g Carbs: 2g Net
Carbs: 2g Fiber: 0g

## 5. Bacon Cheese Pizza

Preparation Time: 5 minutes Cooking Time: 10 minutes
Servings: 2

## Ingredients:

1 cup shredded Mozzarella cheese 1 oz. (28 g) cream cheese, broken into small pieces 4 slices cooked sugar-free bacon, chopped ¼ cup chopped pickled jalapeños 1 large egg, whisked ¼ tsp. salt

## Directions:

Place Mozzarella in a single layer on the bottom of an ungreased 6-inch round nonstick baking dish. Scatter cream cheese pieces, bacon, and jalapeños over Mozzarella, then pour egg evenly around the baking dish. Sprinkle with salt and place into an air fryer basket. Adjust the temperature to 330°F (166°C) and set the timer for 10 minutes. When cheese is brown and egg is set, pizza will be done. Let cool on a large plate 5 minutes before serving. Nutrition: Calories: 361 Fat: 24g Protein: 26g Carbs: 5g Net Carbs: 5g Fiber: 0g

## 6. Bacon-and-Eggs Avocado

Preparation Time: 5 minutes Cooking Time: 17 minutes
Servings: 1

## Ingredients:

1 large egg 1 avocado, halved, peeled, and pitted 2 slices bacon
Fresh parsley, for serving (optional) Sea salt flakes, for garnish
(optional)

## Directions:

Spray the air fryer basket with avocado oil. Preheat the air fryer
to 320°F (160°C). Fill a small bowl with cool water. Soft-boil
the egg: Place the egg in the air fryer basket. Cook for 6 minutes
for a soft yolk or 7 minutes for a cooked yolk. Transfer the egg to
the bowl of cool water and let sit for 2 minutes. Peel and set
aside. Use a spoon to carve out extra space in the center of the
avocado halves until the cavities are big enough to fit the soft-
boiled egg. Place the soft-boiled egg in the center of one half of
the avocado and replace the other half of the avocado on top, so
the avocado appears whole on the outside. Starting at one end
of the avocado, wrap the bacon around the avocado to
completely cover it. Use toothpicks to hold the bacon in place.
Place the bacon-wrapped avocado in the air fryer basket and
cook for 5 minutes. Flip the avocado over and cook for another 5
minutes, or until the bacon is cooked to your liking. Servings on
a bed of fresh parsley, if desired, and sprinkle with salt flakes, if

desired.  Best served fresh. Store extras in an airtight container in the fridge for up to 4 days. Reheat in a preheated 320°F (160°C) air fryer for 4 minutes, or until heated through. Nutrition: Calories: 535 Fat: 46g Protein: 18g Carbs: 18g Net Carbs: 4g Fiber: 14g

---

### 7. Golden Biscuits

Preparation Time: 15 minutes Cooking Time: 13 minutes Servings: 8

**Ingredients:**

2 cups blanched almond flour  ½ cup Swerve confectioners'-style sweetener or equivalent amount of liquid or powdered sweetener  1 tsp. baking powder  ½ tsp. fine sea salt  ¼ cup plus 2 tbsp. (¾ stick) very cold unsalted butter  ¼ cup unsweetened, unflavored almond milk  1 large egg  1 tsp. vanilla extract  3 tsp. ground cinnamon  Glaze: ½ cup Swerve confectioners'-style sweetener or equivalent amount of powdered sweetener  ¼ cup heavy cream or unsweetened, unflavored almond milk

**Directions:**

Preheat the air fryer to 350°F (180°C). Line a pie pan that fits into your air fryer with parchment paper.  In a medium-sized bowl, mix together the almond flour, sweetener (if powdered; do not add liquid sweetener), baking powder, and salt. Cut the butter into ½-inch squares, then use a hand mixer to work the butter into the dry ingredients. When you are done, the mixture should still have chunks of butter. In a small bowl, whisk together the almond milk, egg, and vanilla extract (if using liquid sweetener, add it as well) until blended. Using a fork, stir the wet ingredients into the dry ingredients until large clumps form. Add the cinnamon and use your hands to swirl it into the dough. Form the dough into sixteen 1-inch balls and place them on the prepared pan, spacing them about ½-inch apart. (If you're using a smaller air fryer, work in batches if necessary.) Bake in the air fryer until golden, 10 to 13 minutes. Remove from the air fryer and let cool on the pan for at least 5 minutes. While the biscuits bake, make the glaze: Place the powdered sweetener in a small bowl and slowly stir in the heavy cream with a fork. When the biscuits have cooled somewhat, dip the tops into the glaze, allow it to dry a bit, and then dip again for a thick glaze. Serve warm or at room temperature. Store unglazed biscuits in an airtight container in the refrigerator for up to 3 days or in the freezer for up to a month. Reheat in a preheated 350°F (180°C) air fryer for 5 minutes, or until warmed through, and dip in the glaze as instructed above. Nutrition: Calories: 546 Fat: 51g Protein: 14g Carbs: 13g Net Carbs: 7g Fiber: 6g

## 8. Blueberry Muffin

Preparation Time: 5 minutes Cooking Time: 15 minutes
Servings: 6 Muffins

**Ingredients:**

1½ cups blanched finely ground almond flour  ½ cup granular
erythritol  4 tbsp. salted butter, melted  2 large eggs, whisked  2
tsp. baking powder  1/3 cup fresh blueberries, chopped

**Directions:**

In a large bowl, combine all ingredients. Evenly pour batter
into six silicone muffin cups greased with cooking spray.  Place
muffin cups into air fryer basket. Adjust the temperature to
320°F (160°C) and set the timer for 15 minutes. Muffins should
be golden brown when done.  Let muffins cool in cups for 15
minutes to avoid crumbling. Serve warm.  Nutrition: Calories:
269 Fat: 24g Protein: 8g Carbs: 23g Net Carbs: 20g Fiber: 3g

## 9. Broccoli Frittata

Preparation Time: 15 minutes Cooking Time: 12 minutes
Servings: 4

### Ingredients:

6 large eggs ¼ cup heavy whipping cream ½ cup chopped
broccoli ¼ cup chopped yellow onion ¼ cup chopped green
bell pepper

### Directions:

In a large bowl, whisk eggs and heavy whipping cream. Mix in
broccoli, onion, and bell pepper. Pour into a 6-inch round
oven-safe baking dish. Place baking dish into the air fryer
basket. Adjust the temperature to 350°F (180°C) and set the
timer for 12 minutes. Eggs should be firm and cooked fully
when the frittata is done. Serve warm. Nutrition: Calories: 168
Fat: 11g Protein: 10g Carbs: 3g Net Carbs: 2g Fiber: 1g

# 10. Cauliflower with Avocado

Preparation Time: 15 minutes Cooking Time: 8 minutes Servings: 2

## Ingredients:

1 (12-oz./340-g) steamer bag cauliflower  1 large egg  ½ cup shredded Mozzarella cheese  1 ripe medium avocado  ½ tsp. garlic powder  ¼ tsp. ground black pepper

## Directions:

Cook cauliflower according to package instructions. Remove from bag and place into cheesecloth or clean towel to remove excess moisture.  Place cauliflower into a large bowl and mix in egg and Mozzarella. Cut a piece of parchment to fit your air fryer basket. Separate the cauliflower mixture into two, and place it on the parchment in two mounds. Press out the cauliflower mounds into a ¼-inch-thick rectangle. Place the parchment into the air fryer basket.  Adjust the temperature to 400°F (205°C) and set the timer for 8 minutes.  Flip the cauliflower halfway through the cooking time.  When the timer beeps, remove the parchment and allow the cauliflower to cool for 5 minutes.  Cut open the avocado and remove the pit. Scoop out the inside, place it in a medium bowl, and mash it with garlic powder and pepper. Spread onto the cauliflower. Serve immediately.  Nutrition: Calories: 278 Fat: 15g Protein: 14g Carbs: 16g Net Carbs: 8g Fiber: 8g

## 11. Bacon Calzones

Preparation Time: 15 minutes Cooking Time: 12 minutes
Servings: 4

## Ingredients:

2 large eggs  1 cup blanched finely ground almond flour  2 cups
shredded Mozzarella cheese  2 oz. (57 g) cream cheese, softened
and broken into small pieces  4 slices cooked sugar-free bacon,
crumbled

## Directions:

Beat eggs in a small bowl. Pour into a medium nonstick skillet
over medium heat and scramble. Set aside.  In a large
microwave-safe bowl, mix flour and Mozzarella. Add cream
cheese to the bowl.  Place bowl in the microwave and cook 45
seconds on high to melt cheese, then stir with a fork until a soft
dough ball forms.  Cut a piece of parchment to fit the air fryer
basket. Separate dough into two pieces and press each out into
an 8-inch round.  On half of each dough round, place half of the
scrambled eggs and crumbled bacon. Fold the other side of the
dough over and press to seal the edges.  Place calzones on
ungreased parchment and into an air fryer basket. Adjust the
temperature to 350°F (180°C) and set the timer for 12 minutes,
turning calzones halfway through cooking. The crust will be
golden and firm when done.  Let calzones cool on a cooling rack

5 minutes before serving.  Nutrition: Calories: 477 Fat: 35g Protein: 28g Carbs: 10g Net Carbs: 7g Fiber: 3g

---

## 12. Breakfast Sammies

Preparation Time: 15 minutes Cooking Time: 20 minutes Servings: 5

### Ingredients:

Biscuits: 6 large egg whites  2 cups blanched almond flour, plus more if needed  1½ tsp. baking powder  ½ tsp. fine sea salt  ¼ cup (½ stick) very cold unsalted butter (or lard for dairy-free), cut into ¼-inch pieces  Eggs: 5 large eggs  ½ tsp. fine sea salt  ¼ tsp. ground black pepper  5 (1-oz./28-g) slices Cheddar cheese (omit for dairy-free)  10 thin slices of ham

### Directions:

Spray the air fryer basket with avocado oil. Preheat the air fryer to 350°F (180°C). Grease two 6-inch pie pans or two baking pans that will fit inside your air fryer.  Make the biscuits: In a medium-sized bowl, whip the egg whites with a hand mixer until very stiff. Set aside.  In a separate medium-sized bowl, stir together the almond flour, baking powder, and salt until well combined. Cut in the butter. Gently fold the flour mixture into the egg whites with a rubber spatula. If the dough is too wet to form into mounds, add a few tablespoons of almond flour until the dough holds together well.  Using a large spoon, divide the

16

dough into 5 equal portions and drop them about 1 -inch apart on one of the greased pie pans. (If you're using a smaller air fryer, work in batches if necessary.) Place the pan in the air fryer and cook for 11 to 14 minutes, until the biscuits are golden brown. Remove from the air fryer and set aside to cool.  Make the eggs: Set the air fryer to 375°F (190°C). Crack the eggs into the remaining greased pie pan and sprinkle with salt and pepper. Place the eggs in the air fryer to cook for 5 minutes, or until they are cooked to your liking.  Open the air fryer and top each egg yolk with a slice of cheese (if using). Cook for another minute, or until the cheese is melted.  Once the biscuits are cool, slice them in half lengthwise. Place 1 cooked egg topped with cheese and 2 slices of ham in each biscuit.  Store leftover biscuits, eggs, and ham in separate airtight containers in the fridge for up to 3 days. Reheat the biscuits and eggs on a baking sheet in a preheated 350°F (180°C) air fryer for 5 minutes, or until warmed through.  Nutrition: Calories: 585 Fat: 46g Protein: 36g Carbs: 11g Net Carbs: 6g Fiber: 5g

## 13.Cauliflower Hash Browns

Preparation Time: 20 minutes Cooking Time: 12 minutes Servings: 4

**Ingredients:**

1 (12-oz./340-g) steamer bag cauliflower  1 large egg  1 cup shredded sharp Cheddar cheese

## Directions:

Place bag in the microwave and cook according to package instructions. Allow to cool completely and put cauliflower into a cheesecloth or kitchen towel and squeeze to remove excess moisture. Mash cauliflower with a fork and add egg and cheese. Cut a piece of parchment to fit your air fryer basket. Take ¼ of the mixture and form it into a hash brown patty shape. Place it onto the parchment and into the air fryer basket, working in batches if necessary. Adjust the temperature to 400°F (205°C) and set the timer for 12 minutes. Flip the hash browns halfway through the cooking time. When completely cooked, they will be golden brown. Serve immediately. Nutrition: Calories: 153 Fat: 9g Protein: 10g Carbs: 5g Net Carbs: 3g Fiber: 2g

## 14.Cheesy Danish

Preparation Time: 15 minutes Cooking Time: 20 minutes Servings: 6

## Ingredients:

Pastry: 3 large eggs ¼ tsp. cream of tartar ¼ cup vanilla-flavored egg white protein powder ¼ cup Swerve confectioners'-style sweetener or equivalent amount of liquid or powdered sweetener (see here), or 1 tsp. stevia glycerite 3 tbsp. full-fat sour cream (or coconut cream for dairy-free) 1 tsp. vanilla extract Filling: 4 oz. (113 g) cream cheese (½ cup) (or Kite Hill brand cream cheese style spread for dairy-free), softened  2 large egg yolks (from above)  ¼ cup Swerve confectioners'-style sweetener or equivalent amount of liquid or powdered sweetener, or ½ tsp. stevia glycerite  1 tsp. vanilla extract  ¼ tsp. ground cinnamon  Drizzle: 1 oz. (28 g) cream cheese (2 tbsp.) (or Kite Hill brand cream cheese style spread for dairy-free), softened  1 tbsp. Swerve confectioners'-style sweetener or equivalent amount of liquid or powdered sweetener, or 1 drop of stevia glycerite  1 tbsp. unsweetened, unflavored almond milk (or heavy cream for nut-free)

**Directions:**

Preheat the air fryer to 300°F (150°C). Spray a casserole dish that will fit in your air fryer with avocado oil.  Make the pastry: Separate the eggs putting all the whites in a large bowl, one yolk in a medium-sized bowl, and two yolks in a small bowl. Beat all the egg yolks and set them aside.  Add the cream of tartar to the egg whites. Whip the whites with a hand mixer until very stiff, then turn the hand mixer's setting to low and slowly add the protein powder while mixing. Mix until only just combined; if you mix too long, the whites will fall. Set aside.  To the egg yolk in the medium-sized bowl, add the sweetener, sour cream, and vanilla extract. Mix well. Slowly pour the yolk mixture into the egg whites and gently combine. Dollop 6 equal-sized mounds of batter into the casserole dish. Use the back of a large spoon to make an indentation on the top of each mound. Set aside.  Make the filling: Place the cream cheese in a small bowl and stir to break it up. Add the 2 remaining egg yolks, the sweetener, vanilla extract and cinnamon, and stir until well combined. Divide the filling among the mounds of batter, pouring it into the indentations on the tops. Place the Danish in the air fryer and bake for about 20 minutes, or until golden brown. While the Danish bake, make the drizzle: In a small bowl, stir the cream cheese to break it up. Stir in the sweetener and almond milk. Place the mixture in a piping bag or a small resealable plastic bag with one corner snipped off. After the Danish have cooled, pipe the drizzle over the Danish. Store leftovers in an airtight container in the fridge for up to 4 days. Nutrition: Calories: 160 Fat: 12g Protein: 8g Carbs: 2g Net Carbs: 1g Fiber: 1g

---

## 15. Egg with Cheddar

Preparation Time: 5 minutes Cooking Time: 15 minutes Servings: 2

### Ingredients:

4 large eggs  2 tbsp. unsalted butter, melted  ½ cup shredded sharp Cheddar cheese

### Directions:

 Crack eggs into a 2-cup round baking dish and whisk. Place dish into the air fryer basket. Adjust the temperature to 400°F (205°C) and set the timer for 10 minutes. After 5 minutes, stir the eggs and add the butter and cheese. Let cook for 3 more minutes and stir again. Allow eggs to finish cooking an additional 2 minutes or remove if they are to your desired liking. Use a fork to fluff. Serve warm. Nutrition: Calories: 359 Fat: 27g Protein: 20g Carbs: 1g Net Carbs: 1g Fiber: 0g

## 16. Duo-Cheese Roll

Preparation Time: 10 minutes Cooking Time: 20 minutes Servings: 12 rolls

### Ingredients:

2½ cups shredded Mozzarella cheese  2 oz. (57 g) cream cheese, softened  1 cup blanched finely ground almond flour  ½ tsp. vanilla extract  ½ cup erythritol  1 tbsp. ground cinnamon

**Directions:** In a large microwave-safe bowl, combine Mozzarella cheese, cream cheese, and flour. Microwave the mixture on high for 90 seconds until cheese is melted. Add vanilla extract and erythritol, and mix 2 minutes until a dough form. Once the dough is cool enough to work with your hands, about 2 minutes, spread it out into a 12-inch × 4-inch rectangle on ungreased parchment paper. Evenly sprinkle dough with cinnamon. Starting at the long side of the dough, roll lengthwise to form a log. Slice the log into twelve even pieces. Divide rolls between two ungreased 6-inch round nonstick baking dishes. Place one dish into the air fryer basket. Adjust the temperature to 375°F (190°C) and set the timer for 10 minutes. Cinnamon rolls will be done when golden around the edges and mostly firm. Repeat with the second dish. Allow rolls to cool in dishes 10 minutes before serving.  Nutrition: Calories: 145 Fat: 10g Protein: 8g Carbs: 10g Net Carbs: 9g Fiber: 1g

## 17. Sausage with Peppers

Preparation Time: 15 minutes Cooking Time: 15 minutes Servings: 4

### Ingredients:

½ lb. (227 g) spicy ground pork breakfast sausage  4 large eggs 4 oz. (113 g) full-fat cream cheese, softened  ¼ cup canned diced tomatoes and green chiles, drained  4 large poblano peppers  8 tbsp. shredded pepper jack cheese  ½ cup full-fat sour cream

**Directions:**  In a medium skillet over medium heat, crumble and brown the ground sausage until no pink remains. Remove sausage and drain the fat from the pan. Crack eggs into the pan, scramble, and cook until no longer runny.  Place cooked sausage in a large bowl and fold in cream cheese. Mix in diced tomatoes and chiles. Gently fold in eggs.  Cut a 4-inch–5-inch slit in the top of each poblano, removing the seeds and white membrane with a small knife. Separate the filling into four servings and spoon carefully into each pepper. Top each with 2 tablespoons of pepper jack cheese.  Place each pepper into the air fryer basket.  Adjust the temperature to 350°F (180°C) and set the timer for 15 minutes.  Peppers will be soft and cheese will be browned when ready. Serve immediately with sour cream on top.  Nutrition: Calories: 489 Fat: 35g Protein: 23g Carbs: 13g Net Carbs: 9g Fiber: 4g

## 18.Chocolate Chip Muffin

 Preparation Time: 5 minutes Cooking Time: 15 minutes Servings: 6 Muffins

### Ingredients:

1½ cups blanched finely ground almond flour  1/3 cup granular brown erythritol  4 tbsp. salted butter, melted  2 large eggs, whisked  1 tbsp. baking powder  ½ cup low-carb chocolate chips

### Directions:

In a large bowl, combine all ingredients. Evenly pour batter into six silicone muffin cups greased with cooking spray.  Place muffin cups into air fryer basket. Adjust the temperature to 320°F (160°C) and set the timer for 15 minutes. Muffins will be golden brown when done.  Let muffins cool in cups for 15 minutes to avoid crumbling. Serve warm.  Nutrition: Calories: 329 Fat: 29g Protein: 10g Carbs: 28g Net Carbs: 20g Fiber: 8g

## 19.Simple Ham and Pepper Omelet

Preparation Time: 5 minutes Cooking Time: 8 minutes
Servings: 1

### Ingredients:

2 large eggs ¼ cup unsweetened, unflavored almond milk ¼
tsp. fine sea salt ⅛ tsp. ground black pepper ¼ cup diced ham
(omit for vegetarian) ¼ cup diced green and red bell peppers 2
tbsp. diced green onions, plus more for garnish ¼ cup
shredded Cheddar cheese (about 1 oz./28g) (omit for dairy-free)
Quartered cherry tomatoes, for serving (optional)

### Directions:

Preheat the air fryer to 350°F (180°C). Grease a 6 by 3-inch
cake pan and set it aside.  In a small bowl, use a fork to whisk
together the eggs, almond milk, salt, and pepper. Add the ham,
bell peppers, and green onions. Pour the mixture into the
greased pan. Add the cheese on top (if using).  Place the pan in
the basket of the air fryer. Cook for 8 minutes, or until the eggs
are cooked to your liking.  Loosen the omelet from the sides of
the pan with a spatula and place it on a serving plate. Garnish
with green onions and Servings with cherry tomatoes, if desired.
Best served fresh.  Nutrition: Calories: 476 Fat: 32g Protein: 41g
Carbs: 3g Net Carbs: 2g Fiber: 1g

# FISH AND SEAFOOD

## 20.   Maple Dijon Baked Salmon

Preparation Time: 5 minutes  Cooking Time: 18
minutes  Servings: 5

**Ingredients:**

1½ lbs. salmon  ¼ cup parsley, freshly chopped  ¼ cup Dijon
mustard  1 tbsp. olive oil  1 tsp. maple extract  1 tbsp. freshly-
squeezed lemon juice  1 tbsp. minced garlic  ¼ tsp. salt  ¼ tsp.
ground black pepper

**Directions:**

Preheat your air fryer to 375°F line your air fryer tray with a
piece of parchment paper.   Place the salmon on the parchment-
lined tray.   In a small bowl, mix together the remaining
ingredients and then spread over the top of the salmon.   Place
the salmon in the air fryer and bake for 18 minutes. Slice and
Servings hot!   Nutrition: Calories 254, Total Fat 13 g Saturated
Fat 2 g Total Carbs 2 g Net Carbs 1 g Protein 31 g Sugar 0 g
Fiber 1 g Sodium 373 mg Potassium 42 g

## 21. Creamy Baked Scallops

Preparation Time: 5 minutes  Cooking Time: 5 minutes  Servings: 4

### Ingredients:

1 lb. jumbo scallops  1 tbsp. butter  1 tbsp. heavy cream  ¼ tsp. salt  ¼ tsp. ground black pepper

### Directions:

Preheat your air fryer to 400°F and line your air fryer tray with foil.  Place the butter on the air fryer tray and place inside the air fryer for one minute to melt.  Remove the tray and add the scallops, heavy cream, and seasonings, toss together and return to the air fryer for 5 minutes. The bottom of the scallops should be golden brown.  Servings hot.  Nutrition: Calories 174, Total Fat 10 g Saturated Fat 45 g Total Carbs 3 g Net Carbs 2 g Protein 13 g Sugar 0 g Fiber 1 g Sodium 644 mg Potassium 232 g

## 22. Cajun Seared Scallops

Preparation Time: 5 minutes  Cooking Time: 5 minutes  Servings: 4

**Ingredients:**

1 lb. jumbo scallops  2 tbsp. butter  ½ tsp. Cajun seasoning

**Directions:**

Preheat your air fryer to 400°F and line your air fryer tray with foil.  Place the butter on the air fryer tray and place inside the air fryer for one minute to melt.  Remove the tray and add the scallops and seasonings, toss together and return to the air fryer for 5 minutes. The bottom of the scallops should be golden brown.  Servings hot.  Nutrition: Calories 161, Total Fat 9 g Saturated Fat 4 g Total Carbs 3 g Net Carbs 2 g Protein 13 g Sugar 0 g Fiber 1 g Sodium 627 mg Potassium 230 g

## 23.  Crispy Scallops

Preparation Time: 5 minutes  Cooking Time: 5 minutes  Servings: 4

### Ingredients:

1 lb. jumbo scallops  2 tbsp. butter  ¼ tsp. salt  ¼ tsp. ground black pepper  ¼ cup ground pork rinds

### Directions:

Preheat your air fryer to 400°F and line your air fryer tray with foil.  Place the butter on the air fryer tray and place inside the air fryer for one minute to melt.  Remove the tray and add the scallops, pork rinds, and seasonings, toss together and return to the air fryer for 5 minutes. The bottom of the scallops should be golden brown.  Servings hot.  Nutrition: Calories 182, Total Fat 11 g Saturated Fat 6 g Total Carbs 3 g Net Carbs 2 g Protein 13 g Sugar 0 g Fiber 1 g Sodium 647 mg Potassium 241 g

## 24.   Bacon Scallops

Preparation Time: 5 minutes  Cooking Time: 5 minutes  Servings: 4

## Ingredients:

1 lb. jumbo scallops  1 tbsp. butter  ¼ cup cooked, crumbled bacon  ¼ tsp. salt  ¼ tsp. ground black pepper

## Directions:

Preheat your air fryer to 400°F and line your air fryer tray with foil.  Place the butter on the air fryer tray and place inside the air fryer for one minute to melt.  Remove the tray and add the scallops, bacon and seasonings, toss together and return to the air fryer for 5 minutes. The bottom of the scallops should be golden brown.  Servings hot. Nutrition: Calories 189, Total Fat 12 g Saturated Fat 6 g Total Carbs 3 g Net Carbs 2 g Protein 13 g Sugar 0 g Fiber 1 g Sodium 640 mg Potassium 232 g

## 25. Scallops and Spinach

Preparation Time: 5 minutes  Cooking Time: 5 minutes  Servings: 4

## Ingredients:

1 lb. jumbo scallops  3 cups baby spinach  2 tbsp. butter  ¼ tsp. salt  ¼ tsp. ground black pepper

## Directions:

Preheat your air fryer to 400°F and line your air fryer tray with foil.  Place the butter on the air fryer tray and place inside the air fryer for one minute to melt.  Remove the tray and add the scallops, spinach and seasonings, toss together and return to the air fryer for 5 minutes. The bottom of the scallops should be golden brown.  Servings hot.  Nutrition: Calories 174, Total Fat 9 g Saturated Fat 4 g Total Carbs 5 g Net Carbs 2 g Protein 13 g Sugar 0 g Fiber 3 g Sodium 640 mg Potassium 267 g

## 26.   Salmon and Asparagus

Preparation Time: 20 minutes  Cooking Time: 20 minutes  Servings: 5

### Ingredients:

1¾ lb. salmon fillets   ¼ tsp. salt   ¼ tsp. ground black pepper   3 tbsp. olive oil   1 lb. asparagus spears   1 tbsp. lemon juice   1 tbsp. fresh chopped parsley

### Directions:

Preheat your air fryer to 400°F and line your air fryer tray with a long piece of parchment paper.   Place the salmon fillets on the parchment and sprinkle with salt and pepper and rub the spices into the fish.   Top the fish with the remaining ingredients and then wrap the parchment paper up around the fish fillets, enclosing them completely.   Place the tray in the air fryer and bake for 20 minutes.   Remove from the air fryer, unwrap the parchment, and Servings while hot!   Nutrition: Calories 257, Total Fat 10 g Saturated Fat 4 g Total Carbs 10 g Net Carbs 6 g Protein 33 g Sugar 3 g Fiber 4 g Sodium 492 mg Potassium 325 g

## 27.   Cod and Asparagus

Preparation Time: 20 minutes  Cooking Time: 20 minutes  Servings: 5

### Ingredients:

1¾ lb. cod fillets   ¼ tsp. salt   ¼ tsp. ground black pepper   3 tbsp. olive oil   1 lb. asparagus spears   1 tbsp. lemon juice   1 tbsp. fresh chopped parsley

### Directions:

Preheat your air fryer to 400°F and line your air fryer tray with a long piece of parchment paper.   Place the cod fillets on the parchment and sprinkle with salt and pepper and rub the spices into the fish.   Top the fish with the remaining ingredients and then wrap the parchment paper up around the fish fillets, enclosing them completely.   Place the tray in the air fryer and bake for 20 minutes.   Remove from the air fryer, unwrap the parchment, and Servings while hot!   Nutrition: Calories 235, Total Fat 8 g Saturated Fat 4 g Total Carbs 10 g Net Carbs 6 g Protein 33 g Sugar 3 g Fiber 4 g Sodium 492 mg Potassium 325 g

## 28.  Parmesan Salmon and Asparagus

Preparation Time: 20 minutes  Cooking Time: 20 minutes  Servings: 5

### Ingredients:

1¾ lb. salmon fillets  ¼ tsp. salt  ¼ tsp. ground black pepper  3 tbsp. olive oil  1 lb. asparagus spears  ½ cup grated parmesan cheese  1 tbsp. lemon juice  1 tbsp. fresh chopped parsley

### Directions:

Preheat your air fryer to 400°F and line your air fryer tray with a long piece of parchment paper.   Place the salmon fillets on the parchment and sprinkle with salt and pepper and rub the spices into the fish.   Top the fish with olive oil, asparagus, and lemon juice Sprinkle the parmesan on top along with the parsley.   Place the tray in the air fryer and bake for 20 minutes.   Remove from the air fryer and Servings while hot! Nutrition: Calories 282, Total Fat 14 g Saturated Fat 5 g Total Carbs 11 g Net Carbs 6 g Protein 34 g Sugar 4 g Fiber 4 g Sodium 496 mg Potassium 325 g

## 29.   Parmesan Flounder and Asparagus

Preparation Time: 20 minutes  Cooking Time: 15 minutes  Servings: 5

## Ingredients:

1¾ lbs. flounder fillets   ¼ tsp. salt   ¼ tsp. ground black pepper   3 tbsp. olive oil   1 lb. asparagus spears   ½ cup grated parmesan cheese   1 tbsp. lemon juice   1 tbsp. fresh chopped parsley

## Directions:

Preheat your air fryer to 400°F and line your air fryer tray with a long piece of parchment paper.   Place the flounder fillets on the parchment and sprinkle with salt and pepper and rub the spices into the fish.   Top the fish with olive oil, asparagus, and lemon juice Sprinkle the parmesan on top along with the parsley.   Place the tray in the air fryer and bake for 15 minutes.   Remove from the air fryer and Servings while hot!   Nutrition: Calories 269, Total Fat 13 g Saturated Fat 5 g Total Carbs 11 g Net Carbs 6 g Protein 32 g Sugar 4 g Fiber 4 g Sodium 496 mg Potassium 325 g

## 30.    Parmesan Salmon and Brussel Sprouts

Preparation Time: 20 minutes  Cooking Time: 20 minutes  Servings: 5

### Ingredients:

1¾ lbs. salmon fillets  ¼ tsp. salt  ¼ tsp. ground black pepper  3 tbsp. olive oil  1-lb. sliced Brussel sprouts  ½ cup grated parmesan cheese  1 tbsp. lemon juice  1 tbsp. fresh chopped parsley

### Directions:

Preheat your air fryer to 400°F and line your air fryer tray with a long piece of parchment paper.   Place the salmon fillets on the parchment and sprinkle with salt and pepper and rub the spices into the fish.   Top the fish with olive oil, Brussels sprouts, and lemon juice Sprinkle the parmesan on top along with the parsley. Place the tray in the air fryer and bake for 20 minutes.   Remove from the air fryer and Servings while hot!   Nutrition: Calories 274, Total Fat 13 g Saturated Fat 5 g Total Carbs 11 g Net Carbs 6 g Protein 34 g Sugar 4 g Fiber 4 g Sodium 496 mg Potassium 325 g

## 31. Parmesan Tuna and Brussel Sprouts

Preparation Time: 20 minutes  Cooking Time: 20 minutes  Servings: 5

### Ingredients:

1¾ lbs. tuna fillets   ¼ tsp. salt   ¼ tsp. ground black pepper   3 tbsp. olive oil   1-lb. sliced Brussel sprouts   ½ cup grated parmesan cheese   1 tbsp. lemon juice   1 tbsp. fresh chopped parsley

### Directions:

Preheat your air fryer to 400°F and line your air fryer tray with a long piece of parchment paper.   Place the tuna fillets on the parchment and sprinkle with salt and pepper and rub the spices into the fish.   Top the fish with olive oil, Brussels sprouts, and lemon juice Sprinkle the parmesan on top along with the parsley.   Place the tray in the air fryer and bake for 20 minutes.   Remove from the air fryer and Servings while hot! Nutrition: Calories 285, Total Fat 13 g Saturated Fat 5 g Total Carbs 11 g Net Carbs 6 g Protein 34 g Sugar 4 g Fiber 4 g Sodium 496 mg Potassium 325 g

## 32.  Lemon Dill Wrapped Cod

Preparation Time: 5 minutes  Cooking Time: 15 minutes  Servings: 2

### Ingredients:

1 lb. cod fillets  ¼ tsp. salt  ¼ tsp. ground black pepper  1 tsp. lemon zest  1 tbsp. chopped fresh dill  2 oz. prosciutto di parma, very thinly sliced  2 tbsp. olive oil  1 tsp. minced garlic  4 cups baby spinach  2 tsp. lemon juice

### Directions:

Preheat your air fryer to 325°F and line your air fryer tray with foil.   Dry the cod fillets by patting with a paper towel, sprinkle with salt and pepper.  Sprinkle the lemon zest and dill on the fillets as well.   Wrap the fillets in the prosciutto, enclosing them as fully as possible.   Place the wrapped fillets on the prepared tray.   Toss the spinach with olive oil, garlic and lemon juice and place on the tray as well, around the wrapped cod.   Place in the air fryer and bake for 12 minutes. The spinach should be nicely wilted and the fish 145°F internally.   Servings hot!  Nutrition: Calories 430, Total Fat 20 g Saturated Fat 3 g Total Carbs 11 g Net Carbs 9 g Protein 49 g Sugar 3 g Fiber 2 g Sodium 482 mg Potassium 582 g

## 33.    Mediterranean Salmon

Preparation Time: 20 minutes  Cooking Time: 20 minutes  Servings: 5

## Ingredients:

1¾ lb. salmon fillets  ¼ tsp. salt  1 tsp. smoked paprika  1 tsp. ground dried ginger  ¼ cup pitted olives  ¼ cup sundried tomatoes  ¼ cup capers  1 tbsp. fresh chopped dill  1/3 cup keto pesto sauce

## Directions:

Preheat your air fryer to 400°F and line your air fryer tray with a long piece of parchment paper.   Place the salmon fillets on the parchment and sprinkle with the salt, paprika, and ginger and rub the spices into the fish.   Top the fish with the remaining ingredients and then wrap the parchment paper up around the fish fillets, enclosing them completely.   Place the tray in the air fryer and bake for 20 minutes.   Remove from the air fryer, unwrap the parchment and Servings while hot!   Nutrition: Calories 243, Total Fat 10 g Saturated Fat 4 g Total Carbs 7 g Net Carbs 3 g Protein 33 g Sugar 1 g Fiber 4 g Sodium 489 mg Potassium 321 g

## 34. Lemon Dill Parchment Salmon

Preparation Time: 20 minutes  Cooking Time: 20 minutes  Servings: 5

### Ingredients:

1¾ lbs. salmon fillets  ¼ tsp salt  1 tbsp. fresh chopped dill  1 tsp lemon zest  ¼ cup pitted olives  ¼ cup sundried tomatoes  ¼ cup capers  2 tbsp. olive oil

### Directions:

Preheat your air fryer to 400°F and line your air fryer tray with a long piece of parchment paper.  Place the salmon fillets on the parchment and sprinkle with the salt, lemon zest, and dill and rub the spices into the fish.  Top the fish with the remaining ingredients and then wrap the parchment paper up around the fish fillets, enclosing them completely.  Place the tray in the air fryer and bake for 20 minutes.  Remove from the air fryer, unwrap the parchment, and Servings while hot!  Nutrition: Calories 214, Total Fat 10 g Saturated Fat 4 g Total Carbs 5 g Net Carbs 1 g Protein 33 g Sugar 1 g Fiber 4 g Sodium 489 mg Potassium 321 g

## 35. Mediterranean Flounder

Preparation Time: 20 minutes  Cooking Time: 12 minutes  Servings: 5

### Ingredients:

1¾ lbs. salmon fillets  ¼ tsp. salt  1 tsp. smoked paprika  1 tsp. ground dried ginger  ¼ cup pitted olives  ¼ cup sundried tomatoes  ¼ cup capers  1 tbsp. fresh chopped dill  1/3 cup keto pesto sauce

### Directions:

Preheat your air fryer to 400°F and line your air fryer tray with a long piece of parchment paper.   Place the flounder fillets on the parchment and sprinkle with the salt, paprika, and ginger and rub the spices into the fish.   Top the fish with the remaining ingredients and then wrap the parchment paper up around the fish fillets, enclosing them completely.   Place the tray in the air fryer and bake for 12 minutes.   Remove from the air fryer, unwrap the parchment and Servings while hot!   Nutrition: Calories 211, Total Fat 8 g Saturated Fat 3 g Total Carbs 6 g Net Carbs 3 g Protein 33 g Sugar 1 g Fiber 3 g Sodium 489 mg Potassium 321 g

## 36.    Tomato Parchment Cod

Preparation Time: 20 minutes  Cooking Time: 15 minutes  Servings: 5

### Ingredients:

1¾ lbs. cod fillets  ¼ tsp. salt  1 tsp. smoked paprika  1 tsp. ground dried ginger  ¼ cup pitted olives  ¼ cup sundried tomatoes  ¼ cup capers  1 tbsp. fresh chopped dill  1/3 cup keto marinara

### Directions:

Preheat your air fryer to 400°F and line your air fryer tray with a long piece of parchment paper.   Place the cod fillets on the parchment and sprinkle with the salt, paprika, and ginger and rub the spices into the fish.   Top the fish with the remaining ingredients and then wrap the parchment paper up around the fish fillets, enclosing them completely.   Place the tray in the air fryer and bake for 15 minutes.   Remove from the air fryer, unwrap the parchment, and Servings while hot!   Nutrition: Calories 373, Total Fat 7 g Saturated Fat 3 g Total Carbs 5 g Net Carbs 3 g Protein 33 g Sugar 1 g Fiber 2 g Sodium 489 mg Potassium 321 g

## 37.    Italian Style Flounder

Preparation Time: 20 minutes  Cooking Time: 15 minutes  Servings: 5

### Ingredients:

1¾ lbs. salmon fillets  ¼ tsp. salt  2 tsp. Italian seasoning  1 cup baby spinach  ¼ cup sundried tomatoes  1 tbsp. fresh chopped dill  1/3 cup keto pesto sauce

### Directions:

Preheat your air fryer to 400°F and line your air fryer tray with a long piece of parchment paper.  Place the flounder fillets on the parchment and sprinkle with the salt and Italian seasoning and rub the spices into the fish.  Top the fish with the remaining ingredients and then wrap the parchment paper up around the fish fillets, enclosing them completely.  Place the tray in the air fryer and bake for 20 minutes.  Remove from the air fryer, unwrap the parchment, and Servings while hot!  Nutrition: Calories 226, Total Fat 8 g Saturated Fat 3 g Total Carbs 7 g Net Carbs 3 g Protein 30 g Sugar 2 g Fiber 4 g Sodium 487 mg Potassium 321 g

## 38.  Lemon Parchment Salmon

Preparation Time: 20 minutes  Cooking Time: 20 minutes  Servings: 5

### Ingredients:

1¾ lbs. salmon fillets   ¼ tsp salt   ½ tsp ground black pepper   2 cups baby spinach   1 lemon, sliced thinly

### Directions:

Preheat your air fryer to 400°F and line your air fryer tray with a long piece of parchment paper.   Place the salmon fillets on the parchment and sprinkle with salt and pepper and rub the spices into the fish.   Top the fish with the remaining ingredients and then wrap the parchment paper up around the fish fillets, enclosing them completely.   Place the tray in the air fryer and bake for 20 minutes.   Remove from the air fryer, unwrap the parchment, and Servings while hot!   Nutrition: Calories 264, Total Fat 9 g Saturated Fat 4 g Total Carbs 8 g Net Carbs 3 g Protein 33 g Sugar 1 g Fiber 5 g Sodium 492 mg Potassium 324 g

## 39.   Prosciutto Wrapped Ahi

Preparation Time: 5 minutes  Cooking Time: 20 minutes  Servings: 2

## Ingredients:

1 lb. cod Ahi   ¼ tsp. salt   ¼ tsp. ground black pepper   2 oz. prosciutto di parma, very thinly sliced   2 tbsp. olive oil   1 tsp. minced garlic   4 cups baby spinach   2 tsp. lemon juice

## Directions:

Preheat your air fryer to 325°F and line your air fryer tray with foil.   Dry the cod fillets by patting with a paper towel, sprinkle with salt and pepper.   Wrap the fillets in the prosciutto, enclosing them as fully as possible.   Place the wrapped fillets on the prepared tray.   Place the tray in the air fryer and bake for 10 minutes.   Toss the spinach with olive oil, garlic and lemon juice and remove the tray from the air fryer and place the spinach mix on the tray as well, around the wrapped cod.   Place in the air fryer and bake for another 10 minutes. The spinach should be nicely wilted and the fish 145°F internally.   Servings hot!  Nutrition: Calories 420, Total Fat 20 g Saturated Fat 4 g Total Carbs 11 g Net Carbs 9 g Protein 49 g Sugar 3 g Fiber 2 g Sodium 480 mg Potassium 579 g

# VEGETABLE

### 40.   Vegetable Fried Mix Chips

Preparation Time: 10 minutes  Cooking Time: 35
minutes  Servings: 4

**Ingredients:**

1 large eggplant  4 potatoes  3 zucchinis  ½ cup cornstarch  ½
cup olive oil  Salt to season

**Directions:**

Preheat on Air Fry function to 390°F. Cut the eggplant and
zucchini into long 3-inch strips. Peel and cut the potatoes into
3-inch strips; set aside.   In a bowl, stir in cornstarch, ½ cup of
water, salt, pepper, oil, eggplant, zucchini, and potatoes. Place
one-third of the veggie strips in the basket and fit in the baking
tray; cook for 12 minutes, shaking once.   Once ready, transfer
them to a serving platter. Repeat the cooking process for the
remaining veggie strips. Serve warm.  Nutrition: Calories: 620
Protein: 9.06 g Fat: 27.62 g Carbohydrates: 87.38 g

## 41. Cayenne Spicy Green Beans ccc

Preparation Time: 10 minutes  Cooking Time: 15
minutes  Servings: 4

### Ingredients:

1 cup panko breadcrumbs  2 whole eggs, beaten  ½ cup
Parmesan cheese, grated  ½ cup flour  1 tsp. cayenne pepper
1½ lbs. green beans  Salt to taste

### Directions:

In a bowl, mix panko breadcrumbs, Parmesan cheese, cayenne
pepper, salt, and pepper. Roll the green beans in flour and dip
them in eggs.  Dredge beans in the parmesan-panko mix. Place
the prepared beans in the greased cooking basket and fit in the
baking tray; cook for 15 minutes on Air Fry function at 350°F,
shaking once. Serve and enjoy!  Nutrition: Calories: 213 Protein:
11.61 g Fat: 9.31 g Carbohydrates: 21.77 g

## 42.   Cheesy Cabbage Wedges

Preparation Time: 5 minutes  Cooking Time: 20 minutes  Servings: 4

### Ingredients:

½ head cabbage, cut into wedges   2 cups Parmesan cheese, chopped   4 tbsp. melted butter  Salt and black pepper to taste  ½ cup blue cheese sauce

### Directions:

Brush the cabbage wedges with butter and coat with mozzarella cheese.  Place the coated wedges in the greased basket and fit in the baking tray; cook for 20 minutes at 380°F on Air Fry setting. Serve with blue cheese sauce. Nutrition: Calories: 398 Protein: 18.71 g Fat: 30.11 g Carbohydrates: 14.92 g

## 43. Traditional Jacket Potatoes

Preparation Time: 10 minutes  Cooking Time: 20
minutes  Servings: 4

**Ingredients:**

Four potatoes, well washed  Two garlic cloves, minced  Salt and
black pepper to taste  1 tsp. rosemary  1 tsp. butter

**Directions:**

Preheat your Oven to 360°F on the Air Fry function. Prick the
potatoes with a fork.   Put them into your Air fryer basket and fit
in the baking tray; cook for 25 minutes. Cut the potatoes in half
and top with butter and rosemary; season with salt and pepper.
Serve immediately.  Nutrition: Calories: 300 Protein: 7.79 g Fat:
1.33 g Carbohydrates: 66.06 g

## 44.   Garlicky Veggie Bake

Preparation Time: 5 minutes  Cooking Time: 15 minutes  Servings: 3

### Ingredients:

3 turnips, sliced  1 large red onion, cut into rings  1 large zucchini, sliced   Salt and black pepper to taste  2 cloves garlic, crushed  1 bay leaf, cut into six pieces  1 tbsp. olive oil

### Directions:

Place the turnips, onion, and zucchini in a bowl. Toss with olive oil, salt, and pepper.  Preheat on Air Fry function to 380°F. Places the veggies into a baking pan. Slip the bay leaves into the slices' different parts and tuck the garlic cloves between the slices. Cook for 15 minutes. Serve warm with as a side to a meat dish or salad.   Nutrition: Calories: 68 Protein: 1.75 g Fat: 4.89 g Carbohydrates: 5.62 g

## 45. Sweet Baby Carrots

Preparation Time: 5 minutes  Cooking Time: 15 minutes  Servings: 4

**Ingredients:**

1 lb. baby carrots  1 tsp. dried dill  1 tbsp. olive oil  1 tbsp. honey Salt and black pepper to taste

**Directions:**

Preheat your Oven to 300°F on the Air Fry function. In a bowl, mix oil, carrots, and honey; gently stir to coat.  Season with dill, pepper, and salt. Place the carrots in the cooking basket and fit in the baking tray; cook for 15 minutes, shaking once. Serve.  Nutrition: Calories: 92 Protein: 1.05 g Fat: 3.62 g Carbohydrates: 15.02 g

## 46.   Colorful Vegetarian Delight

Preparation Time: 5 minutes  Cooking Time: 16 minutes  Servings: 2

### Ingredients:

One parsnip, sliced in a 2-inch thickness  1 cup chopped butternut squash   Two small red onions, cut into wedges  1 cup chopped celery  1 tbsp. chopped fresh thyme  Salt and black pepper to taste  2 tsp. olive oil

### Directions:

Preheat on Air Fry function to 380°F.  In a bowl, add turnip, squash, red onions, celery, thyme, pepper, salt, and olive oil; mix well. Add the veggies to the basket and fit in the baking tray; cook for 16 minutes, tossing once halfway through. Serve. Nutrition: Calories: 167 Protein: 3.13 g Fat: 4.99 g Carbohydrates: 30.61 g

### 47.  Awesome Sweet Potato Fries

Preparation Time: 10 minutes  Cooking Time: 20 minutes  Servings: 4

### Ingredients:

½ tsp. salt  ½ tsp. garlic powder  ½ tsp. chili powder  ¼ tsp. cumin  3 tbsp. olive oil  3 sweet potatoes, cut into thick strips

### Directions:

In a bowl, mix salt, garlic powder, chili, and cumin, and olive oil. Coat the strips well in this mixture and arrange them in the basket without overcrowding.  Fit in the baking tray and cook for 20 minutes at 380°F on Air Fry function or until crispy. Serve.  Nutrition: Calories: 92 Protein: 0.14 g Fat: 10.21 g Carbohydrates: 0.52 g

## 48.    Rosemary Butternut Squash Roast

Preparation Time: 10 minutes  Cooking Time: 20 minutes  Servings: 2

### Ingredients:

1 butternut squash   1 tbsp. dried rosemary   2 tbsp. maple syrup Salt to taste

### Directions:

Put the squash on a cutting board and peel. Cut in half and remove the seeds and pulp. Slice into wedges and season with salt.   Preheat on Air Fry function to 350°F. Spray the wedges with cooking spray and sprinkle with rosemary. Place the wedges in the basket without overlapping and fit in the baking tray. Cook for 20 minutes, until halfway through, turning. Serve with maple syrup and goat cheese.   Nutrition: Calories: 53 Protein: 0.04 g Fat: 0.06 g Carbohydrates: 13.58 g

## 49.   Cheesy Frittata with Vegetables

Preparation Time: 5 minutes  Cooking Time: 20 minutes  Servings: 2

### Ingredients:

1 cup baby spinach  1/3 cup sliced mushrooms  1 zucchini, sliced with a 1-inch thickness  1 small red onion, sliced   ¼ cup chopped chives  ¼ lb. asparagus, trimmed and sliced thinly  2 tsp. olive oil  4 eggs, cracked into a bowl  1/3 cup milk  Salt and black pepper to taste  1/3 cup grated Cheddar cheese  1/3 cup crumbled Feta cheese

### Directions:

Preheat on the Bake function to 320°F. Line a baking dish with parchment paper. Mix the beaten eggs with milk, salt, and pepper.  Heat olive oil in a skillet over medium heat adds stir-fry asparagus, zucchini, onion, mushrooms, and baby spinach for 5 minutes. Pour the veggies into the baking dish and top with the egg mixture. Sprinkle with feta and cheddar cheeses. Cook for 15 minutes. Garnish with chives.  Nutrition: Calories: 429 Protein: 25.5 g Fat: 30.61 g Carbohydrates: 13.57 g

## 50.    Cauliflower Rice with Tofu & Peas

Preparation Time: 10 minutes  Cooking Time: 22 minutes  Servings: 4

### Ingredients:

Tofu: ½ block tofu, crumbled  ½ cup diced onion  2 tbsp. soy sauce  1 tsp. turmeric  1 cup diced carrot  Cauliflower: 3 cups cauliflower rice  2 tbsp. soy sauce  ½ cup chopped broccoli  2 garlic cloves, minced  1½ tsp. toasted sesame oil  1 tbsp. minced ginger  ½ cup frozen peas  1 tbsp. rice vinegar

### Directions:

Preheat on Air Fry function to 370°F. Combine all the tofu ingredients in a greased baking dish. Cook for 10 minutes.  Meanwhile, place all cauliflower ingredients in a large bowl and mix to combine. Stir the cauliflower mixture in the tofu baking dish, return to the oven; cook for 12 minutes. Serve. Nutrition: Calories: 409 Protein: 18.02 g Fat: 25.38 g Carbohydrates: 55.7 g

## 51. Chickpea & Carrot Balls

Preparation Time: 5 minutes  Cooking Time: 20 minutes  Servings: 3

### Ingredients:

2 tbsp. olive oil  2 tbsp. soy sauce  1 tbsp. flax meal  2 cups cooked chickpeas  ½ cup sweet onions  ½ cup grated carrots  ½ cup roasted cashews  Juice of 1 lemon  ½ tsp. turmeric  1 tsp. cumin  1 tsp. garlic powder  1 cup rolled oats

### Directions:

Combine the olive oil, onions, and carrots into the Air Fryer baking pan and cook them on the Air Fry function for 6 minutes at 350°F. Ground the oats and cashews in a food processor. Place in a large bowl. Mix in the chickpeas, lemon juice, and soy sauce.  Add onions and carrots to the bowl with chickpeas. Stir in the remaining ingredients; mix until fully incorporated. Make meatballs out of the mixture. Increase the temperature to 370°F and cook for 12 minutes.  Nutrition: Calories: 500 Protein: 16.62 g Fat: 29.24 g Carbohydrates: 56.41 g

## 52.   Yummy Chili Bean Burritos

Preparation Time: 10 minutes  Cooking Time: 20 minutes  Servings: 3

### Ingredients:

6 tortillas  1 cup grated cheddar cheese   One can (8 oz.) of beans  1 tsp. Italian seasoning

### Directions:

Preheat on the Bake function to 350°F. Season the beans with the seasoning and divide them between the tortillas.   Top with cheddar cheese. Roll the burritos and arrange them on a lined baking dish. Cook for 5 minutes. Serve.  Nutrition: Calories: 279 Protein: 7.52 g Fat: 5.53 g Carbohydrates: 48.76 g

## 53.   Tasty Polenta Crisps

Preparation Time: 5 minutes  Cooking Time: 16 minutes  Servings: 4

### Ingredients:

2 cups of milk  1 cup instant polenta  Salt and black pepper to taste  fresh thyme, chopped

### Directions:

Fill a saucepan with milk and 2 cups of water and place over low heat. Bring to a simmer. Keep whisking as you pour in the polenta.   Continue to whisk until polenta thickens and bubbles; season to taste. Add polenta to a lined with parchment paper baking tray and spread out.   Refrigerate for 45 minutes. Slice set polenta into batons, and spray with olive oil. Arrange polenta chips into the basket and fit in the baking tray; cook for 16 minutes at 380°F on Air Fry function, turning once halfway through. Make sure that the fries are golden and crispy. Serve. Nutrition: Calories: 121 Protein: 5.53 g Fat: 4.07 g Carbohydrates: 15.94 g

## 54.  Garlicky Fennel Cabbage Steaks

Preparation Time: 10 minutes  Cooking Time: 15 minutes  Servings: 3

## Ingredients:

1 cabbage head  1 tbsp. garlic paste  1 tsp. salt  2 tbsp. olive oil ½ tsp. black pepper  2 tsp. fennel seeds

## Directions:

Preheat on Air Fry function to 350°F. Slice the cabbage into one ½-inch slice. In a prepared small bowl, combine all the other ingredients; brush cabbage with the mixture.  Arrange the steaks on a greased baking dish and cook for 15 minutes, flipping once. Serve.  Nutrition: Calories: 148 Protein: 3.15 g Fat: 9.53 g Carbohydrates: 15.88 g

## 55.  Simple Ricotta & Spinach Balls

Preparation Time: 5 minutes  Cooking Time: 12 minutes  Servings: 4

### Ingredients:

14 oz. store-bought crescent dough  1 cup steamed spinach  1 cup crumbled ricotta cheese  ¼ tsp. garlic powder  1 tsp. chopped oregano  ¼ tsp. salt

### Directions:

Preheat on Air Fry function to 350°F. Rolls the dough onto a lightly floured flat surface. Combine the ricotta cheese, spinach, oregano, salt, and garlic powder in a bowl. Cut the dough into four equal pieces.  Divide the spinach/feta mixture between the dough pieces. Make sure to place the filling in the center. Fold the dough and secure it with a fork. Place onto a lined baking dish and then in your oven. Cook for 12 minutes until lightly browned. Serve.  Nutrition: Calories: 135 Protein: 8.45 g Fat: 8.27 g Carbohydrates: 7.8 g

## 56.   Baby Spinach & Pumpkin with Nuts & Cheese

Preparation Time: 10 minutes  Cooking Time: 25 minutes  Servings: 1

### Ingredients:

½ small pumpkin  2 oz. blue cheese, crumbled  2 tbsp. pine nuts 1 tbsp. olive oil  ½ cup baby spinach, packed  1 spring onion, sliced  1 radish, thinly sliced  1 tsp. vinegar

### Directions:

Preheat on Toast function to 330°F. Place the pine nuts in the Air Fryer pan and toast them for 5 minutes; set aside. Peel the pumpkin and then chop it into small pieces and toss them with olive oil. Place in the Air Fryer basket and fit in the baking tray. Increase the temperature to 390°F and cook for 20 minutes.   Remove the pumpkin to a serving bowl. Add in baby spinach, radish, and spring onion; toss with the vinegar. Stir in the blue cheese and top with the toasted pine nuts to serve. Nutrition: Calories: 413 Protein: 17.48 g Fat: 30.9 g Carbohydrates: 20.01 g

## 57.Mom's Blooming Buttery Onion

Preparation Time: 10 minutes  Cooking Time: 30 minutes  Servings: 4

**Ingredients:**

4 onions  2 tbsp. butter, melted  1 tbsp. olive oil

**Directions:**

Preheat on Air Fry function to 350°F. Peel the onions and slice off the root bottom so it can sit well. Cut slices into the onion to make it look like a blooming flower, make sure not to go all the way through; four cuts will do.  Place the onions in a greased baking tray. Drizzle with olive oil and butter and cook for about 30 minutes. Serve with garlic mayo dip.  Nutrition: Calories: 125 Protein: 1.27 g Fat: 9.24 g Carbohydrates: 10.28 g

## 58.    Mozzarella Eggplant Patties

Preparation Time: 5 minutes  Cooking Time: 7
minutes  Servings: 1

### Ingredients:

1 hamburger bun  1 eggplant, sliced  1 mozzarella slice, chopped
1 red onion cut into three rings  1 lettuce leaf  ½ tbsp. tomato
sauce  1 pickle, sliced

### Directions:

Preheat on the Bake function to 330°F. Place the eggplant slices
in a greased baking tray and cook for 6 minutes. Take out the
tray and top the eggplant with mozzarella cheese and cook for
30 more seconds.  Spread tomato sauce on one half of the bun.
Place the lettuce leaf on top of the sauce. Place the cheesy
eggplant on top of the lettuce. Top with onion rings and pickles
and then with the other bun half to serve.  Nutrition: Calories:
823 Protein: 63.05 g Fat: 34.05 g Carbohydrates: 69.87 g

## 59. Sandwiches with Tomato, Nuts & Cheese

Preparation Time: 10 minutes  Cooking Time: 42 minutes  Servings: 2

### Ingredients:

1 heirloom tomato  1 (4-oz.) block feta cheese  1 small red onion, thinly sliced  1 clove garlic  Salt to taste  2 tsp. + ¼ cup olive oil  1½ tbsp. toasted pine nuts  ¼ cup chopped parsley  ¼ cup grated Parmesan cheese  ¼ cup chopped basil

### Directions:

Add basil, pine nuts, garlic, and salt to a food processor. Process while slowly adding ¼ cup of olive oil. Once finished, pour basil pesto into a bowl and refrigerate for 30 minutes.  Preheat on Air Fry function to 390°F. Slice the feta cheese and tomato into ½-inch slices. Remove the pesto from the fridge and spread half of it on the tomato slices. Top with feta cheese slices and onion. Drizzle the remaining olive oil on top.  Place the tomatoes in the fryer basket and fit in the baking tray; cook for 12 minutes. Remove to a serving platter and top with the remaining pesto. Serve.  Nutrition: Calories: 1977 Protein: 4.63 g Fat: 219.77 g Carbohydrates: 4.57 g

## 60. Roasted Butternut Squash

Preparation Time: 10 minutes Cooking Time: 35 to 40 minutes  Servings: 4

### Ingredients:

3 lbs. butternut squash, peeled, seeded, and cut into 1-inch cubes  ½ tsp. cinnamon  1½ tbsp. maple syrup  1½ tbsp. olive oil  Pepper  Salt

### Directions:

Line roasting pan with parchment paper and set aside.  Insert wire rack in rack position 6. Select roast, set temperature 400°F, timer for 40 minutes. Press start to preheat the oven.  In a mixing bowl, toss squash cubes with the remaining ingredients.  Spread squash cubes in a prepared roasting pan. Roast squash cubes for 35-40 minutes.  Serve and enjoy. Nutrition: Calories 219 Fat 5.6 g Carbohydrates 45.1 g Sugar 12 g Protein 3.4 g

# 61.Cholesterol 0 mg Oven Roasted Broccoli

Preparation Time: 10 minutes Cooking Time: 25 minutes  Servings: 4

## Ingredients:

1½ lbs. broccoli florets  1 tbsp. fresh lemon juice  ¼ tsp. onion powder  ½ tsp. garlic powder  2½ tbsp. olive oil  ¼ tsp. pepper  ½ tsp. salt

## Directions:

Line roasting pan with parchment paper and set aside.  Insert wire rack in rack position 6. Select bake, set temperature 390°F, timer for 25 minutes. Press start to preheat the oven.  In a bowl, toss broccoli with onion powder, garlic powder, olive oil, pepper, and salt.  Spread broccoli florets on a roasting pan and bake for 25 minutes or until tender.  Drizzle lemon juice over broccoli and serve.  Nutrition: Calories 136 Fat 9.3 g Carbohydrates 11.8 g Sugar3.1 g Protein 4.9 g Cholesterol 0 mg

# MEAT

## 62.   Carne Asada Tacos

Preparation Time: 5 minutes Cooking Time: 14 minutes
Servings: 4

### Ingredients:

1/3 cup olive oil  1½ lbs. (680 g) flank steak  Salt and freshly
ground black pepper, to taste  1/3 cup freshly squeezed lime
juice  ½ cup chopped fresh cilantro  4 tsp. minced garlic  1 tsp.
ground cumin  1 tsp. chili powder

### Directions:

Brush the air fryer basket with olive oil.  Put the flank steak in a
large mixing bowl. Season with salt and pepper.  Add the lime
juice, cilantro, garlic, cumin, and chili powder and toss to coat
the steak.  For the best flavor, let the steak marinate in the
refrigerator for about 1 hour.  Preheat the air fryer to 400°F
(204°C)  Put the steak in the air fryer basket. Air fry for 7
minutes. Flip the steak. Air fry for 7 minutes more or until an
internal temperature reaches at least 145°F (63°C).  Let the
steak rest for about 5 minutes, then cut into strips to serve.
Nutrition: Calories: 734 Protein: 37.11 g Fat: 62.79 g
Carbohydrates: 6.66 g

## 63.  Air Fried Baby Back Ribs

Preparation Time: 5 minutes Cooking Time: 30 minutes
Servings: 2

### Ingredients:

2 tsp. red pepper flakes   ¾ ground ginger   3 cloves minced
garlic   Salt and ground black pepper, to taste   2 baby back ribs

### Directions:

Preheat the air fryer to 350°F (177°C).  Combine the red pepper
flakes, ginger, garlic, salt and pepper in a bowl, making sure to
mix well. Massage the mixture into the baby back ribs.  Air fry
the ribs in the air fryer for 30 minutes.  Take care when taking
the rubs out of the air fryer. Put them on a serving dish and
serve.  Nutrition: Calories: 3486 Protein: 309.51 g Fat: 245.86 g
Carbohydrates: 11 g

## 64.  Bacon-Wrapped Pork with Apple Gravy

Preparation Time: 10 minutes Cooking Time: 25 minutes
Servings: 4

### Ingredients:

Pork: 1 tbsp. Dijon mustard  1 pork tenderloin  3 strips bacon
Apple Gravy: 3 tbsp. ghee, divided  1 small shallot, chopped  2
apples  1 tbsp. almond flour  1 cup vegetable broth  ½ tsp. Dijon
mustard

### Directions:

Preheat the air fryer to 360°F (182°C).  Spread Dijon mustard
all over tenderloin and wrap with strips of bacon.  Put into an
air fryer and air fry for 12 minutes. Use a meat thermometer to
check for doneness.  To make sauce, heat 1 tablespoons of ghee
in a pan and add shallots. Cook for 1 minute.  Then add apples,
cooking for 4 minutes until softened.   Add flour and 2
tablespoons of ghee to make a roux. Add broth and mustard,
stirring well to combine.  When the sauce starts to bubble, add 1
cup of sautéed apples, cooking until sauce thickens.  Once pork
tenderloin is cooked, allow to sit 8 minutes to rest before
slicing.  Serve topped with apple gravy.  Nutrition: Calories: 68
Protein: 0.93 g Fat: 1.57 g Carbohydrates: 14.3 g

## 65.   Bacon and Pear Stuffed Pork Chops

Preparation Time: 20 minutes Cooking Time: 24 minutes
Servings: 3

### Ingredients:

4 slices bacon, chopped  1 tbsp. butter  ½ cup finely diced onion
1/3 cup chicken stock  1½ cups seasoned stuffing cubes  1 egg,
beaten  ½ tsp. dried thyme  ½ tsp. salt  ⅛ tsp. freshly ground
black pepper  1 pear, finely diced  1/3 cup crumbled blue cheese
3 boneless center-cut pork chops (2-inch thick)  Olive oil, for
greasing  Salt and freshly ground black pepper, to taste

### Directions:

Preheat the air fryer to 400°F (204°C).  Put the bacon into the
air fryer basket and air fry for 6 minutes, stirring halfway
through the cooking time. Remove the bacon and set it aside on
a paper towel. Pour out the grease from the bottom of the air
fryer.  To make the stuffing, melt the butter in a medium
saucepan over medium heat on the stovetop. Add the onion and
sauté for a few minutes until it starts to soften. Add the chicken
stock and simmer for 1 minute. Remove the pan from the heat
and add the stuffing cubes. Stir until the stock has been
absorbed. Add the egg, dried thyme, salt and freshly ground
black pepper, and stir until combined. Fold in the diced pear
and crumbled blue cheese.  Put the pork chops on a cutting
board. Using the palm of the hand to hold the chop flat and

steady, slice into the side of the pork chop to make a pocket in the center of the chop. Leave about an inch of chop uncut and make sure you don't cut all the way through the pork chop. Brush both sides of the pork chops with olive oil and season with salt and freshly ground black pepper. Stuff each pork chop with a third of the stuffing, packing the stuffing tightly inside the pocket. Preheat the air fryer to 360°F (182°C). Spray or brush the sides of the air fryer basket with oil. Put the pork chops in the air fryer basket with the open, stuffed edge of the pork chop facing the outside edges of the basket. Air fry the pork chops for 18 minutes, turning the pork chops over halfway through the cooking time. When the chops are done, let them rest for 5 minutes and then transfer to a serving platter. Nutrition: Calories: 768 Protein: 41.5 g Fat: 40.28 g Carbohydrates: 46 g

## 66.    Kale and Beef Omelet

Preparation Time: 15 minutes Cooking Time: 16 minutes Servings: 4

## Ingredients:

½ lb. (227 g) leftover beef, coarsely chopped   2 garlic cloves, pressed   1 cup kale, torn into pieces and wilted   1 tomato, chopped   ¼ tsp. sugar   4 eggs, beaten   4 tbsp. heavy cream   ½ tsp. turmeric powder   Salt and ground black pepper, to taste   ⅛ tsp. ground allspice   Cooking spray

## Directions:

Preheat the air fryer to 360°F (182°C). Spritz four ramekins with cooking spray. Put equal amounts of each of the ingredients into each ramekin and mix well. Air fry for 16 minutes. Serve immediately. Nutrition: Calories: 430 Protein: 28.9 g Fat: 29.85 g Carbohydrates: 11.21g

---

## 67.  Spinach and Beef Braciole

Preparation Time: 25 minutes Cooking Time: 1 hour 32 minutes Servings: 4

## Ingredients:

½ onion, finely chopped  1 tsp. olive oil  $1/3$ cup red wine  2 cups crushed tomatoes  1 tsp. Italian seasoning  ½ tsp. garlic powder  ¼ tsp. crushed red pepper flakes  2 tbsp. chopped fresh parsley  2 top round steaks (about 1½ lbs./680 g)  salt and freshly ground black pepper  2 cups fresh spinach, chopped  1 clove minced garlic  ½ cup roasted red peppers, julienned  ½ cup grated pecorino cheese  ¼ cup pine nuts, toasted and roughly chopped  2 tbsp. olive oil

## Directions:

Preheat the air fryer to 400°F (204°C). Toss the onions and olive oil together in a baking pan or casserole dish. Air fry at 400°F (204°C) for 5 minutes, stirring a couple of times during the cooking process. Add the red wine, crushed tomatoes,

Italian seasoning, garlic powder, red pepper flakes and parsley and stir. Cover the pan tightly with aluminum foil, lower the air fryer temperature to 350°F (177°C) and continue to air fry for 15 minutes. While the sauce is simmering, prepare the beef. Using a meat mallet, pound the beef until it is ¼-inch thick. Season both sides of the beef with salt and pepper. Combine the spinach, garlic, red peppers, pecorino cheese, pine nuts and olive oil in a medium bowl. Season with salt and freshly ground black pepper. Disperse the mixture over the steaks. Starting at one of the short ends, roll the beef around the filling, tucking in the sides as you roll to ensure the filling is completely enclosed. Secure the beef rolls with toothpicks. Remove the baking pan with the sauce from the air fryer and set it aside. Preheat the air fryer to 400°F (204°C). Brush or spray the beef rolls with a little olive oil and air fry at 400°F (204°C) for 12 minutes, rotating the beef during the cooking process for even browning. When the beef is browned, submerge the rolls into the sauce in the baking pan, cover the pan with foil and return it to the air fryer. Reduce the temperature of the air fryer to 250°F (121°C) and air fry for 60 minutes. Remove the beef rolls from the sauce. Cut each roll into slices and serve, ladling some sauce over top. Nutrition: Calories: 442 Protein: 46.33 g Fat: 22.59 g Carbohydrates: 10.21 g

## 68. Beef and Cheddar Burgers

Preparation Time: 20 minutes Cooking Time: 25 minutes
Servings: 4

### Ingredients:

1 tbsp. olive oil 1 onion, sliced into rings 1 tsp. garlic, minced or puréed 1 tsp. mustard 1 tsp. basil 1 tsp. mixed herbs Salt and ground black pepper, to taste 1 tsp. tomato, puréed 4 buns 1 oz. (28 g) Cheddar cheese, sliced 10 oz. (298 g) beef, minced Salad leaves

### Directions:

Preheat the air fryer to 390°F (199°C). Grease the air fryer with olive oil and allow it to warm up. Put the diced onion in the air fryer and air fry until they turn golden brown. Mix in the garlic, mustard, basil, herbs, salt, and pepper, and air fry for 25 minutes. Lay 2 to 3 onion rings and puréed tomato on two of the buns. Put one slice of cheese and the layer of beef on top. Top with salad leaves before closing off the sandwich with the other buns. Serve immediately. Nutrition: Calories: 443 Protein: 19.53 g Fat: 25.64 g Carbohydrates: 34.1 g

## 69. Beef and Pork Sausage Meatloaf

Preparation Time: 20 minutes Cooking Time: 25 minutes
Servings: 4

### Ingredients:

¾ lb. (340 g) ground chuck  4 oz. (113 g) ground pork
sausage  1 cup shallots, finely chopped  2 eggs, well beaten  3
tbsp. plain milk  1 tbsp. oyster sauce  1 tsp. porcini
mushrooms  ½ tsp. cumin powder  1 tsp. garlic paste  1 tbsp.
fresh parsley  Salt and crushed red pepper flakes, to taste  1 cup
crushed saltines  Cooking spray

### Directions:

Preheat the air fryer to 360°F (182°C). Spritz a baking dish with
cooking spray.  Mix all the ingredients in a large bowl,
combining everything well.  Transfer to the baking dish and
bake in the air fryer for 25 minutes.  Serve hot.  Nutrition:
Calories: 385 Protein: 29.32 g Fat: 21.08 g Carbohydrates: 19.35
g

## 70. Beef and Spinach Rolls

Preparation Time: 10 minutes Cooking Time: 14 minutes
Servings: 2

### Ingredients:

3 tsp. pesto   2 lbs. (907 g) beef flank steak   6 slices provolone
cheese   3 oz. (85 g) roasted red bell peppers   ¾ cup baby
spinach   1 tsp. sea salt   1 tsp. black pepper

### Directions:

Preheat the air fryer to 400°F (204°C).  Spoon equal amounts
of the pesto onto each flank steak and spread it across
evenly.  Put the cheese, roasted red peppers and spinach on top
of the meat, about three-quarters of the way down.  Roll the
steak up, holding it in place with toothpicks. Sprinkle with sea
salt and pepper.  Put inside the air fryer and air fry for 14
minutes, turning halfway through the cooking time.  Allow the
beef to rest for 10 minutes before slicing up and
serving.  Nutrition: Calories: 940 Protein: 115.27 g Fat: 44.51 g
Carbohydrates: 14.27 g

### 71. Beef Egg Rolls

Preparation Time: 15 minutes Cooking Time: 12 minutes
Servings: 8 egg rolls

## Ingredients:

½ chopped onion  2 garlic cloves, chopped  ½ packet taco
seasoning   Salt and ground black pepper, to taste  1 lb. (454 g)
lean ground beef   ½ can cilantro lime rotel  16 egg roll
wrappers  1 cup shredded Mexican cheese  1 tbsp. olive oil  1
tsp. cilantro

## Directions:

Preheat the air fryer to 400°F (205°C).  Add onions and garlic
to a skillet, cooking until fragrant. Then add taco seasoning,
pepper, salt, and beef, cooking until beef is broke up into tiny
pieces and cooked thoroughly.  Add rotel and stir well.  Lay out
egg wrappers and brush with a touch of water to soften a bit.
Load wrappers with beef filling and add cheese to each.  Fold
diagonally to close and use water to secure edges.  Brush filled
egg wrappers with olive oil and add to the air fryer.  Air fry 8
minutes, flip, and air fry for another 4 minutes.  Serve sprinkled
with cilantro.  Nutrition: Calories: 383 Protein: 25 g Fat: 12.97 g
Carbohydrates: 39.88 g

## 72. Peppercorn Crusted Beef Tenderloin

Preparation Time: 5 minutes Cooking Time: 25 minutes

Servings: 6

### Ingredients:

2 lbs. (907 g) beef tenderloin   2 tsp. roasted garlic, minced   2 tbsp. salted butter, melted   3 tbsp. ground 4-peppercorn blender

### Directions:

Preheat the air fryer to 400°F (204°C).  Remove any surplus fat from the beef tenderloin.  Combine the roasted garlic and melted butter to apply to the tenderloin with a brush.  On a plate, spread out the peppercorns and roll the tenderloin in them, making sure they are covering and clinging to the meat.  Air fry the tenderloin in the air fryer for 25 minutes, turning halfway through cooking.  Let the tenderloin rest for ten minutes before slicing and serving.  Nutrition: Calories: 343 Protein: 46.2 g Fat: 16.02 g Carbohydrates: 0.31 g

## 73.  Pork Chops with Rinds

Preparation Time: 5 minutes Cooking Time: 15 minutes

Servings: 4

### Ingredients:

1 tsp. chili powder  ½ tsp. garlic powder  1½ oz. (43 g) pork rinds, finely ground  4 (4-oz./113-g) pork chops  1 tbsp. coconut oil, melted

### Directions:

Preheat the air fryer to 400°F (204°C).  Combine the chili powder, garlic powder, and ground pork rinds.  Coat the pork chops with coconut oil, followed by the pork rind mixture, taking care to cover them completely. Then place the chops in the air fryer basket.  Air fry the chops for 15 minutes or until the internal temperature of the chops reaches at least 145°F (63°C), turning halfway through.  Serve immediately.
Nutrition: Calories: 389 Protein: 43.03 g Fat: 22.74 g
Carbohydrates: 0.63 g

## 74. Beef Chuck with Brussels Sprouts

Preparation Time: 20 minutes Cooking Time: 15 minutes
Servings: 4

### Ingredients:

1 lb. (454 g) beef chuck shoulder steak   2 tbsp. vegetable oil   1
tbsp. red wine vinegar   1 tsp. fine sea salt   ½ tsp. ground black
pepper   1 tsp. smoked paprika   1 tsp. onion powder   ½ tsp.
garlic powder   ½ lb. (227 g) Brussels sprouts, cleaned and
halved   ½ tsp. fennel seeds   1 tsp. dried basil   1 tsp. dried sage

### Directions:

Massage the beef with vegetable oil, wine vinegar, salt, black
pepper, paprika, onion powder, and garlic powder, coating it
well.   Allow to marinate for a minimum of 3 hours.   Preheat the
air fryer to 390°F (199°C).   Remove the beef from the marinade
and put in the preheated air fryer. Air fry for 10 minutes. Flip
the beef halfway through.   Put the prepared Brussels sprouts in
the air fryer along with the fennel seeds, basil, and sage.   Lower
the heat to 380°F (193°C) and air fry everything for another 5
minutes.   Give them a good stir. Air fry for an additional 10
minutes.   Serve immediately.   Nutrition: Calories: 252 Protein:
26.3 g Fat: 13.38 g Carbohydrates: 7.01 g

## 75.BBQ Pork Steaks

Preparation Time: 5 minutes Cooking Time: 15 minutes
Servings: 4

### Ingredients:

4 pork steaks 1 tbsp. Cajun seasoning 2 tbsp. BBQ sauce 1
tbsp. vinegar 1 tsp. soy sauce ½ cup brown sugar ½ cup
ketchup

### Directions:

Preheat the air fryer to 290°F (143°C). Sprinkle pork steaks
with Cajun seasoning. Combine remaining ingredients and
brush onto steaks. Add coated steaks to the air fryer. Air fry 15
minutes until just browned. Serve immediately. Nutrition:
Calories: 643 Protein: 47.05 g Fat: 33.01 g Carbohydrates: 37.41
g

## 76.    Cheddar Bacon Burst with Spinach

Preparation Time: 5 minutes Cooking Time: 60 minutes
Servings: 8

### Ingredients:

30 slices bacon  1 tbsp. Chipotle seasoning  2 tsp. Italian
seasoning  2½ cups Cheddar cheese  4 cups raw spinach

### Directions:

Preheat the air fryer to 375°F (191°C).  Weave the bacon into 15
vertical pieces and 12 horizontal pieces. Cut the extra 3 in half to
fill in the rest, horizontally.  Season the bacon with Chipotle
seasoning and Italian seasoning.  Add the cheese to the
bacon.  Add the spinach and press down to compress.  Tightly
roll up the woven bacon.  Line a baking sheet with kitchen foil
and add plenty of salt to it.  Put the bacon on top of a cooling
rack and put that on top of the baking sheet.  Bake for 60
minutes.  Let cool for 15 minutes before slicing and serve.
Nutrition: Calories: 406 Protein: 12.73 g Fat: 38.35 g
Carbohydrates: 2.39 g

## 77. Beef Cheeseburger Egg Rolls

Preparation Time: 15 minutes Cooking Time: 8 minutes
Servings: 6 egg rolls

### Ingredients:

8 oz. (227 g) raw lean ground beef ½ cup chopped onion ½
cup chopped bell pepper ¼ tsp. onion powder ¼ tsp. garlic
powder 3 tbsp. cream cheese 1 tbsp. yellow mustard 3 tbsp.
shredded Cheddar cheese 6 chopped dill pickle chips 6-egg roll
wrappers

### Directions:

Preheat the air fryer to 392°F (200°C). In a skillet, add the
beef, onion, bell pepper, onion powder, and garlic powder. Stir
and crumble beef until fully cooked, and vegetables are soft.
Take the skillet off the heat and add cream cheese, mustard, and
Cheddar cheese, stirring until melted. Pour beef mixture into a
bowl and fold in pickles. Lay out egg wrappers and divide the
beef mixture into each one. Moisten egg roll wrapper edges with
water. Fold sides to the middle and seal with water. Repeat
with all other egg rolls. Put rolls into an air fryer, one batch at a
time. Air fry for 8 minutes. Serve immediately. Nutrition:
Calories: 211 Protein: 14.08 g Fat: 6.96 g Carbohydrates: 21.95 g

## 78.    Beef Chuck Cheeseburgers

Preparation Time: 10 minutes Cooking Time: 15 minutes

Servings: 4

### Ingredients:

¾ lb. (340 g) ground beef chuck   1 envelope onion soup
mix   Kosher salt and freshly ground black pepper, to taste   1
tsp. paprika   4 slices Monterey Jack cheese   4 ciabatta rolls

### Directions:

In a bowl, stir together the ground chuck, onion soup mix, salt,
black pepper, and paprika to combine well.   Preheat the air
fryer to 385°F (196°C).   Take four equal portions of the mixture
and mold each one into a patty. Transfer to the air fryer and air
fry for 10 minutes.   Put the slices of cheese on the top of the
burgers.  Air fry for another minute before serving on ciabatta
rolls.   Nutrition: Calories: 336 Protein: 28.53 g Fat: 14.99 g
Carbohydrates: 21.56 g

## 79.    Chicken Fried Steak

Preparation Time: 15 minutes Cooking Time: 10 minutes

Servings: 4

### Ingredients:

½ cup flour  2 tsp. salt, divided  Freshly ground black pepper, to
taste  ¼ tsp. garlic powder  1 cup buttermilk  1 cup fine bread

crumbs  4 (6-oz./170-g) tenderized top round steaks, ½-inch thick  Vegetable or canola oil  For the Gravy: 2 tbsp. butter or bacon drippings  ¼ onion, minced  1 clove garlic, smashed  ¼ tsp. dried thyme  3 tbsp. flour  1 cup milk  Salt and freshly ground black pepper, to taste  Dashes of Worcestershire sauce

## Directions:

Set up a dredging station. Combine the flour, 1 teaspoon of salt, black pepper and garlic powder in a shallow bowl. Pour the buttermilk into a second shallow bowl. Finally, put the bread crumbs and 1 teaspoon of salt in a third shallow bowl.  Dip the tenderized steaks into the flour, then the buttermilk, and then the bread crumb mixture, pressing the crumbs onto the steak. Put them on a baking sheet and spray both sides generously with vegetable or canola oil.  Preheat the air fryer to 400°F (204°C).  Transfer the steaks to the air fryer basket, two at a time, and air fry for 10 minutes, flipping the steaks over halfway through the cooking time. Hold the first batch of steaks warm in a 170°F (77°C) oven while you air fry the second batch.  While the steaks are cooking, make the gravy. Melt the butter in a small saucepan over medium heat on the stovetop. Add the onion, garlic and thyme and cook for five minutes, until the onion is soft and just starting to brown. Stir in the flour and cook for another five minutes, stirring regularly, until the mixture starts to brown. Whisk in the milk and bring the mixture to a boil to thicken. Season to taste with salt, lots of freshly ground black pepper, and a few dashes of Worcestershire sauce. Pour the gravy over the chicken fried steaks and serve. Nutrition: Calories: 654 Protein: 87.05 g Fat: 19.16 g Carbohydrates: 27.61 g

## 80.    Super Bacon with Meat

Preparation Time: 1 hour 25 minutes Cooking Time: 1 hour Servings: 4

**Ingredients:** 30 slices thick-cut bacon  4 oz. (113 g) Cheddar cheese, shredded  12 oz. (340 g) steak  10 oz. (283 g) pork sausage  Salt and ground black pepper, to taste

**Directions:** Preheat the air fryer to 400°F (204°C).  Lay out 30 slices of bacon in a woven pattern and bake for 20 minutes until crisp. Put the cheese in the center of the bacon.  Combine the steak and sausage to form a meaty mixture.  Lay out the meat in a rectangle of similar size to the bacon strips. Season with salt and pepper.  Roll the meat into a tight roll and refrigerate.  Preheat the air fryer to 400°F (204°C).  Make a 7×7 bacon weave and roll the bacon weave over the meat, diagonally.  Bake for 60 minutes or until the internal temperature reaches at least 165°F (74°C).  Let rest for 5 minutes before serving.  Nutrition: Calories: 1178 Protein: 59.35 g Fat: 101.47 g Carbohydrates: 6.5 g

## 81.Sun-Dried Tomato Crusted Chops

Preparation Time: 15 minutes Cooking Time: 10 minutes

Servings: 4

### Ingredients:

½ cup oil-packed sun-dried tomatoes ½ cup toasted almonds ¼ cup grated Parmesan cheese ½ cup olive oil, plus more for brushing the air fryer basket 2 tbsp. water ½ tsp. salt Freshly ground black pepper, to taste 4 center-cut boneless pork chops (about 1¼ lbs./567 g)

### Directions:

Put the sun-dried tomatoes into a food processor and pulse them until they are coarsely chopped. Add the almonds, Parmesan cheese, olive oil, water, salt and pepper. Process into a smooth paste. Spread most of the paste (leave a little in reserve) onto both sides of the pork chops and then pierce the meat several times with a needle-style meat tenderizer or a fork. Let the pork chops sit and marinate for at least 1 hour (refrigerate if marinating for longer than 1 hour). Preheat the air fryer to 370°F (188°C). Brush more olive oil on the bottom of the air fryer basket. Transfer the pork chops into the air fryer basket, spooning a little more of the sun-dried tomato paste onto the pork chops if there are any gaps where the paste may have been rubbed off. Air fry the pork chops for 10 minutes, turning the chops over halfway through. When the pork chops have finished cooking, transfer them to a serving plate and serve.  Nutrition: Calories: 295 Protein: 2.5 g Fat: 30.75 g Carbohydrates: 4.11 g

## 82.   Pork Wellington

Preparation Time: 20 minutes Cooking Time: 30 minutes Servings: 6

### Ingredients:

1½ lb. pork tenderloin  ½ tsp. salt  ½ tsp. pepper  1 tsp. thyme 1 sheet puff pastry  4 oz. prosciutto, sliced thin  1 tbsp. Dijon mustard  1 tbsp. olive oil  1 tbsp. butter  8 oz. mushrooms, chopped  1 shallot, chopped  1 egg, beaten

### Directions:

 Season tenderloin with salt, pepper, and thyme on all sides.  On parchment-covered work surface, roll out the pastry as long as the tenderloin and wide enough to cover it completely.  Lay the prosciutto across the pastry to cover it and spread with mustard. Melt butter and oil in a large skillet over high heat. Add mushrooms and shallot and cook 5-10 minutes, until golden brown. Remove from pan.  Add tenderloin to the skillet and brown on all sides.  Spread mushrooms over the mustard and add pork. Roll up to completely cover tenderloin. Use beaten egg to seal the edge.  Set oven to bake on 425°F for 35 minutes. Line baking pan with parchment paper and place pork on it, seam side down. Brush top with remaining egg. After the oven preheats for 5 minutes, place pan in position 1 and cook for 30 or until puffed and golden brown. Remove from oven and let rest 5 minutes before slicing and serving. Nutrition: Calories: 457, Total Fat 25 g Saturated Fat 7 g Total Carbs 20 g Net Carbs 19 g Protein 38 g Sugar 1 g Fiber 1g

# DESSERT

### 83. Biscuits

Preparation Time: 10 minutes Cooking Time: 25 minutes
Servings: 6 biscuits

## Ingredients:

2 cups of all-purpose flour ¾ cup of 2% or full-fat milk, very
cold 6 tbsp. of unsalted butter, very cold 2½ tsp. of baking
powder 1 tsp. of salt 1 tsp. of sugar

## Directions:

Preheat your air fryer to 390°F. Spray the inside of the basket
with some oil. Add flour, salt, sugar, and baking powder to a
medium bowl. Mix it well. Cut butter into small pieces and add
into the flour mixture. Pour in milk and mix until fully
combined. Take the dough out and put it on the floured work
surface. Press dough with your hands into a rectangle. Fold the
dough a couple of times, then flatten it until you reach a 1-inch-
thick layer. Using around a 3-inch biscuit cutter, make 6
biscuits from the dough. Put them in the preheated air fryer in
a single layer. Avoid touching each other. Cook at 390°F for 9–
11 minutes until golden-brown crispy. Remove and brush with
some melted butter. Serve and enjoy your Biscuits! Nutrition:
Calories: 275 Carbohydrates: 35 g Fat: 13 g Protein: 5 g Sugar: 2
g Sodium: 405 mg Cholesterol: 33mg

## 84.  Churros

Preparation Time: 10 minutes Cooking Time: 90 minutes
Servings: 6

### Ingredients:

1 cup of all-purpose flour  1 cup of water  2 large eggs  1/3 cup
of unsalted butter  ½ cup + 2 tbsp. of granulated sugar  1 tsp. of
vanilla exact  ¾ tsp. of ground cinnamon  ¼ tsp. of salt

### Directions:

Place a silicone baking mat on a baking sheet. Grease it with
some oil.  Add sugar, salt, butter, and water to a saucepan. Bring
to a boil, then reduce to medium-low heat.  Add flour into the
saucepan. Using a rubber spatula, stir it constantly until the
smooth dough. Remove from the heat and put in a mixing bowl.
Let it rest for 5 minutes.  Add vanilla extract and eggs into the
bowl with the dough. Mix it with a hand mixer until smooth
consistency. The dough texture will look like gluey mashed
potatoes. Press the dough into a ball and put it into a large
piping bag with a large star-shaped tip at the end.  Squeeze 4-
inch lengths churros out on the oiled baking mat. Cut the end
with the scissors. Keep in a refrigerator for 1 hour.  Preheat your
air fryer to 375°F. Spray the inside of the basket with some oil.
Gently put churros into the air fryer basket, leaving some space
around them. Cook at 375°F for 10–12 minutes until golden-
brown crispy.  Meanwhile, mix the cinnamon with granulated

sugar in a shallow dish. Remove churros from the air fryer and coat with the sugar mixture. Serve warm with the chocolate sauce Nutella. Enjoy your Churros! Nutrition: Calories: 204 Carbohydrates: 27 g Fat: 9 g Protein: 3 g Sugar: 15 g Sodium: 91 mg Cholesterol: 61mg

## 85. Donuts

Preparation Time: 10 minutes Cooking Time: 120 minutes Servings: 14 donuts

### Ingredients:

3 cups of all-purpose flour 1 cup of milk, warmed to around 110°F 4 tbsp. of unsalted melted butter 1 large egg ¼ cup +1 tsp. of sugar 2½ tsp. of active dry yeast ½ tsp. of kosher salt For Glaze: 2 cups of powdered sugar 6 tbsp. of unsalted melted butter 2 tsp. of vanilla extract 2–4 tbsp. of hot water

### Directions:

Add the warm milk, yeast, and 1 teaspoon of sugar to a large bowl. Stir it for 5–10 minutes until foamy. Add the egg, ¼ cup of sugar, and salt into the milk mixture. Stir it until combined. Pour in the melted butter with 2 cups of flour and mix. Scrape the sides of the bowl down, and add in 1 more cup of flour. Mix it well until the dough starts pulling away from the bowl but leaves sticky. Continue kneading for 5–10 minutes. Cover the bowl with plastic wrap. Leave it for 30 minutes until the dough doubled. Spread some flour on the work surface. Transfer the dough onto it and roll into a ½-¼-inch-thick layer. Cut out donuts with a round cutter (about 3 inches in diameter). Use a smaller cutter (about 1 inch in diameter) and cut out the centers. Transfer the formed donuts onto the oiled parchment paper, and cover them with oiled plastic wrap. Leave it for 20–30 minutes until the dough is doubled. Preheat your air fryer to 350°F. Spray the inside of the basket with some oil. Put the formed donuts in the preheated air fryer in a single layer. Avoid them touching. Lightly spray tops with oil. Cook at 350°F for 4–5 minutes. Repeat this step with the remaining part of donuts and their holes. For making glaze: Meantime, pour the melted butter into a medium bowl. Add in vanilla and powdered sugar. Whisk until combined. Stir in 1 tablespoon of hot water at a time until you reach the desired consistency. After cooling the cooked donuts for a few minutes, glaze them until fully coated. Put donuts on the rack to drip off the excess of the glaze until it hardens. Serve and enjoy your Donuts! Nutrition: Calories: 270 Carbohydrates: 32 g Fat: 14 g Protein: 3 g Sugar: 17 g Sodium: 70 mg Cholesterol: 25mg

## 86.  S'mores

Preparation Time: 10 minutes Cooking Time: 15 minutes
Servings: 4 s'mores

### Ingredients:

4 marshmallows  4 graham crackers, divided in half  1 milk chocolate, divided

### Directions:

Put 4 halves of graham crackers into the air fryer basket.  Cut off a small piece from the bottom of each marshmallow and put the marshmallow on the crackers, which will help to stick them well.  Cook at 375°F for 7–8 minutes until golden-brown.  Add on the top the pieces of chocolate and cover with another half of crackers.  Continue cooking for about 2 minutes until the chocolate starts melting.  Serve and enjoy your S'mores!
Nutrition: (1 S'more): Calories: 152 Carbohydrates: 25 g Fat: 5.5 g Protein: 2.2 g Sugar: 16.2 g Sodium: 102 mg Cholesterol: 4 mg

## 87.  Chocolate Lava Cake

Preparation Time: 10 minutes Cooking Time: 25 minutes Servings: 6

### Ingredients:

8 oz. of baking chocolate bar (about 60% cacao)  3 egg yolks  3 large eggs  1½ cups of powdered sugar  ½ cup of all-purpose flour  10 tbsp. of unsalted butter  ½ tsp. of salt

### Directions:

Preheat your air fryer to 400°F.  Grease with some oil 6 oven-safe 6-ounce ramekins.  Divide the chocolate into small pieces and put them into a medium bowl. Add in butter. Put in a microwave on medium heat power for 90 seconds, stirring every 30 seconds, until you reach a smooth consistency.  Add in flour, sugar, and salt. Mix it until well combined.   Whisk in eggs and egg yolks. Your batter should become thick but still pourable. Pour all the prepared batter into the ramekins. Put as many ramekins as it can stand in your air fryer basket.  Cook at 400°F for 8 minutes (for a runny center) or 10 minutes (for a thicker one). Remove from the basket and leave it for at least 2 minutes. Serve warm and enjoy your Chocolate Lava Cake!  Nutrition: (1 Serving): Calories: 510 Carbohydrates: 62 g Fat: 29 g Protein: 7 g Sugar: 48 g Sodium: 290 mg Cholesterol: 200mg

## 88.  Chocolate Chip Cookies

Preparation Time: 10 minutes Cooking Time: 40 minutes
Servings: 10 cookies

### Ingredients:

1 cup of all-purpose flour ¼ cup of rolled oats 1 cup of semi-sweet chocolate chips ½ cup of chopped walnuts 1/3 cup of brown sugar 1/3 cup of granulated sugar 8 tbsp. of softened butter 1 large egg 1 tsp. of vanilla extract ½ tsp. of salt ½ tsp. of baking soda ¼ tsp. of cinnamon ⅛ tsp. of lemon juice

### Directions:

Blend brown sugar, granulated sugar, and butter in a mixing bowl using a hand or stand mixer for 2 minutes.  Pour in lemon juice, vanilla, and egg. Blend it on low speed for 30 seconds. Then mix on medium speed for 2–3 minutes until fluffy consistency.  Mix in on low-speed oats, flour, cinnamon, baking soda, and salt; blend for 45–60 seconds. Fold in walnuts and chocolate chips.  Preheat your air fryer to 300°F. Cover the inside of the air fryer basket with a piece of parchment paper. Take about 2 tablespoons of the dough and shape a ball. Put in the preheated air fryer basket around 1½ to 2 inches apart. Flatten the tops of the cookies with wet hands.  Cook at 300°F for 6–8 minutes. Remove and cool for about 5 minutes before taking the cookies out, otherwise, they can crumble.  Repeat the last 2 steps with the remaining cookies.  Serve and enjoy your

Chocolate Chip Cookies! Nutrition: Calories: 353
Carbohydrates: 39 g Fat: 20.1 g Protein: 5.4 g Sugar: 24.3 g
Cholesterol: 43 mg

---

## 89.   Gluten-Free Chocolate Cake

Preparation Time: 10 minutes Cooking Time: 1 hour 15 minutes
Servings: 10

### Ingredients:

1 cup of almond flour  2/3 cup of sugar  3 large eggs  1/3 cup of
heavy cream  ¼ cup of unsweetened cocoa powder  ¼ cup of
melted coconut oil  ⅛ cup of chopped pecans  ⅛ cup of
chopped walnuts  1 tsp. of baking powder  ½ tsp. of orange zest
Unsalted butter, for greasing

### Directions:

Take a 7-inch round baking pan, cover the bottom with
parchment paper and grease it with unsalted butter.  Put all the
ingredients into a large mixing bowl. Blend the mixture on
medium speed using a hand mixer until you receive the fluffy
and light batter.  Gently fold in the walnuts and pecans.
Transfer the prepared batter into the baking pan and cover it
with a piece of aluminum foil.  Put the baking pan into the air
fryer basket. Cook at 325°F for 45 minutes. Take the foil out and
cook for extra 10–15 minutes until done. To check the readiness,
insert the toothpick in the center; it should come out clean.

Remove the pan from the air fryer. Let it cool for 10 minutes. Then take the cooked cake out from the pan and allow it to cool for extra 20 minutes. Serve with berries and enjoy your Gluten-Free Chocolate Cake! Nutrition: Calories: 232 Carbohydrates: 17 g Fat: 17 g Protein: 4 g Sugar: 13 g Sodium: 22 mg Cholesterol: 59 mg

---

## 90. Apple Crisp

Preparation Time: 10 minutes Cooking Time: 30 minutes Servings: 2

### Ingredients:

2 chopped apples  3 tbsp. of old fashioned oats  4 tbsp. of brown sugar  2½ tbsp. of flour  2 tbsp. of cold butter  1 tsp. of lemon juice  1 tsp. of cinnamon  Pinch of salt

### Directions:

Preheat your air fryer to 400°F. Grease with some butter an oven-safe 5-inch oval baking dish.  Cut apples into small cubes into a bowl. Add in sugar, cinnamon, and lemon juice. Mix and transfer it into the baking pan.  Cover the dish with a piece of aluminum foil and put it in the preheated air fryer basket. Cook at 400°F for 15 minutes. Remove the foil and continue cooking for an extra 5 minutes.  Meanwhile, put flour, oatmeal, cold butter, salt, and sugar into the mixer with the paddle attachment. Blend on low speed until you receive the crumbly mixture. Open the basket and spread the prepared oatmeal mixture over the apples. Cook for additional 5 minutes until lightly brown. Serve* warm and enjoy your Apple Crisp. Nutrition: Calories: 384 Carbohydrates: 67 g Fat: 13 g Protein: 3.7 g Sugar: 41.2 g Cholesterol: 31 mg

---

## 91.Fried Oreos

Preparation Time: 10 minutes Cooking Time: 20 minutes Servings: 12 cookies

### Ingredients:

12 Oreos or other chocolate sandwich cookies  1 cup of pancake and baking mix  ¼ cup of milk  1 large egg  2 tbsp. of sugar  1 tsp. of vanilla extract

### Directions:

Cover the air fryer basket with a piece of parchment paper and spray some oil over it. Preheat your air fryer to 350°F. Add the milk, vanilla, and egg to a medium bowl. Whisk it until mix. Add in the pancake mix and sugar, continue whisking. The batter consistency should be thick, just to coat the cookie. Take 6 cookies and dip them in the prepared batter, wait until excess will drip back. Place the coated cookies in the preheated air fryer basket in a single layer. Avoid touching each other! Cook at 350°F for about 7 minutes until golden-brown. Repeat the last step with the remaining part of the cookies. Top with some powdered sugar. Serve and enjoy your Fried Oreos! Nutrition: Calories: 355 Carbohydrates: 61.5 g Fat: 13 g Protein: 3.3 g Sugar: 37.5 g

---

## 92.   Blueberry Muffins

Preparation Time: 10 minutes Cooking Time: 35 minutes Servings: 3

### Ingredients:

1 egg  2/3 cup of flour  ½ cup of blueberries*  1/3 cup of oil  1/3 cup of sugar  2 tbsp. of water  1 tsp. of lemon zest  ½ tsp. of baking powder  ¼ tsp. of vanilla extract  Pinch of salt

### Directions:

Preheat your air fryer to 350°F.  Add the egg, oil, water, and vanilla to a medium bowl. Whisk until smooth consistency.  Mix the sugar, lemon zest, flour, baking powder, and salt in a separate bowl. Add the dry ingredients into the wet ones. Stir until smooth.  Gently fold in the blueberries.  Cover oven-safe 1-cup ramekins with muffin papers. Put the prepared batter into each ramekin. Cook at 350°F for 15–17 minutes.  Serve and enjoy your Blueberry Muffins! Nutrition: Calories: 39 Carbohydrates: 1 g Fat: 3 g Protein: 2 g Sugar: 1 g Sodium: 68 mg Cholesterol: 62 mg

## 93.  Baklava Purses

Preparation Time: 10 minutes Cooking Time: 25 minutes
Servings: 4

### Ingredients:

4 stacks of 8 sheets of phyllo dough (4x4 inches)  1 egg  ¼ cup
of chopped walnuts  1 tbsp. of chopped pistachios  2 tbsp. of
melted butter  1 tsp. of honey  Cinnamon, to taste  Orange zest,
to taste

### Directions:

Preheat your air fryer to 375°F. Grease the inside of the air fryer
basket with some oil.  Grease every second sheet of the phyllo
dough with the melted butter. Place the chopped walnuts in the
center, then pour the honey on them, and sprinkle some orange
zest and cinnamon.  Press the corners together and push down
into the honey to stick them and made it look like a "purse." Put
the prepared baklava in the preheated air fryer. Cook at 375°F
for 6–8 minutes until golden-brown crispy. Top with the
chopped pistachios.  Repeat the last 2 steps until all dough is
used.  Serve with honey and enjoy your Baklava Purses!
Nutrition: Calories: 311 Carbohydrates: 30 g Fat: 21 g Protein: 2
g Sodium: 281 mg Cholesterol: 15 mg

## 94.  Apple Turnovers

Preparation Time: 10 minutes Cooking Time: 45 minutes
Servings: 4

### Ingredients:

2 diced medium Granny Smith apples  6 tbsp. of brown sugar
¼ cup of powdered sugar  ½ package pastry (14 oz.) for crust
pie  4 tbsp. of butter  1 tsp. of cornstarch  1 tsp. of ground
cinnamon  1 tsp. of milk  2 tsp. of cold water  ½ tbsp. of oil

### Directions:

Put the diced apples, cinnamon, brown sugar, and butter into a
non-stick skillet. Cook on medium heat for 5 minutes until it
softened.  Dissolve the cornstarch in cold water. Pour it into the
apples and cook for 1 minute until it thickened. Remove it from
the heat and allow cooling.  Spread some flour over the work
surface, place the dough on it, and roll it out. Cut the rolled
dough into rectangles small enough so that 2 can fit in the air
fryer at a time. You should make 8 equal rectangles at the end.
Put some apple mixture in the center of the rectangles, about
½-inch from each edge. Roll out the other 4 rectangles to make
them slightly larger than the filled ones. Put the larger
rectangles on the top of the fillings and push the edges down
with a fork to stick. Make small cuts in the center of the tops of
the pies. Grease the tops with oil.  Preheat your air fryer to
385°F. Grease the inside of the air fryer basket with some oil.

Place the prepared pies into the preheated air fryer basket. Cook at 385°F for about 8 minutes until golden-brown. Remove them out and cook the other part of the pies. Whisk milk with powdered sugar in a small bowl. Glaze the warm pies with the milk-sugar mixture. Serve warm and enjoy your Apple Turnovers! Nutrition: Calories: 497 Carbohydrates: 59.7 g Fat: 28.6 g Protein: 3.2 g Sodium: 327 mg Cholesterol: 30.5 mg

## 95. Chocolaty Banana Muffins

Preparation Time: 5 minutes  Cooking Time: 25 minutes Servings: 12

### Ingredients:

¾ cup whole wheat flour  ¾ cup plain flour  ¼ cup cocoa powder  ¼ tsp. baking powder  1 tsp. baking soda  ¼ tsp. salt  2 large bananas, peeled and mashed  1 cup sugar  1/3 cup canola oil  1 egg  ½ tsp. vanilla essence  1 cup mini chocolate chips

### Directions:

Preparing the Ingredients. In a large bowl, mix together flour, cocoa powder, baking powder, baking soda, and salt.  In another bowl, add bananas, sugar, oil, egg and vanilla extract and beat till well combined.  Slowly, add flour mixture in egg mixture and mix till just combined.  Fold in chocolate chips.  Preheat the Air Fryer to 345°F. Grease 12 muffin molds.   Air Frying. Transfer the mixture into prepared muffin molds evenly and cook for about 20-25 minutes or till a toothpick inserted in the center comes out clean.   Remove the muffin molds from Air fryer and keep on a wire rack to cool for about 10 minutes. Carefully turn on a wire rack to cool completely before serving.   Nutrition: Calories 75 Fat 6.5g Protein 1.7g Sugar 2g

## 96.   Black and White Brownies

Preparation Time: 10 minutes  Cooking Time: 20 minutes Servings: 8

### Ingredients:

1 egg   ¼ cup brown sugar   2 tbsp. white sugar   2 tbsp. safflower oil   1 tsp. vanilla   ¼ cup cocoa powder   1/3 cup all-purpose flour   ¼ cup white chocolate chips   Nonstick baking spray with flour

### Directions:

Preparing the Ingredients. In a medium bowl, beat the egg with brown sugar and white sugar. Beat in the oil and vanilla.   Add the cocoa powder and flour, and stir just until combined. Fold in the white chocolate chips.   Spray a 6-by-6-by-2-inch baking pan with nonstick spray. Spoon the brownie batter into the pan.   Air Frying. Bake for 20 minutes or until the brownies are set when lightly touched with a finger. Let cool for 30 minutes

before slicing to serve.   Nutrition:  Calories 81 Fat 4g Protein 1g
Fiber 1g

## 97.    Baked Apple

Preparation Time: 5 minutes  Cooking Time: 20 minutes
Servings: 4

### Ingredients:

¼ cup water    ¼ tsp. nutmeg    ¼ tsp. cinnamon    1½ tsp.
melted ghee    2 tbsp. raisins    2 tbsp. chopped walnuts    1
medium apple

### Directions:

Preparing the ingredients. Preheat your air fryer to
350°F.    Slice an apple in half and discard some of the flesh
from the center.    Place into a frying pan.    Mix remaining
ingredients together except water. Spoon mixture to the middle
of apple halves.    Pour water overfilled apples.    Air Frying.
Place pan with apple halves into the Air Fryer Oven, bake 20
minutes.    Nutrition:  Calories 199 Fat 9g Protein 1g Sugar 3g

## 98.   Cinnamon Fried Bananas

Preparation Time: 5 minutes  Cooking Time: 10 minutes

Servings: 2-3

### Ingredients:

1 cup panko breadcrumbs    3 tbsp. cinnamon    ½ cup almond flour    3 egg whites    8 ripe bananas    3 tbsp. vegan coconut oil

### Directions:

Preparing the Ingredients. Heat coconut oil and add breadcrumbs. Mix around 2-3 minutes until golden. Pour into a bowl.    Peel and cut bananas in half. Roll the hall of each banana into flour, eggs, and crumb mixture.   Air Frying. Place into the Air Fryer Oven. Cook 10 minutes at 280°F.    A great addition to a healthy banana split!    Nutrition:  Calories 219 Fat 10g Protein 3g Sugar 5g

## 99.  Awesome Chinese Doughnuts

 Preparation Time: 10 minutes  Cooking Time: 8 minutes
Servings: 8

### Ingredients:

 1 tbsp. baking powder  6 tbsp. Coconut oil  ¾ cup of coconut
milk  2 tsp. Sugar  2 cup all-purpose flour  ½ tsp. sea salt

### Directions:

Preheat the air fryer to 350°F.  Mix baking powder, flour, sugar,
and salt in a bowl.  Add coconut oil and mix well. Add coconut
milk and mix until well combined.  Knead the dough for 3-4
minutes.  Roll dough half-inch thick and using a cookie cutter
cut doughnuts.  Place doughnuts in cake pan and brush with
oil. Place cake pan in the air fryer basket and air fry doughnuts
for 5 minutes. Turn doughnuts to another side and air fry for 3
minutes more.  Serve and enjoy.  Nutrition: Calories 259 Fat
15.9g Carbohydrates 27g Protein 3.8g

## 100.  Crispy Bananas

Preparation Time: 10 minutes  Cooking Time: 10 minutes
Servings: 4

### Ingredients:

4 sliced ripe bananas   1 egg   ½ cup breadcrumbs   1½ tbsp.
Cinnamon sugar   1 tbsp. almond meal   1½ tbsp. Coconut oil   1
tbsp. crushed cashew   ¼ cup corn flour

### Directions:

Set the pan on fire to heat the coconut oil over medium heat and
add breadcrumbs in the pan and stir for 3-4 minutes.  Remove
pan from heat and transfer breadcrumbs to a bowl.  Add
almond meal and crush cashew in breadcrumbs and mix
well.  Dip banana half in corn flour then in egg and finally coat
with breadcrumbs.  Place coated banana in the air fryer basket.
Sprinkle with Cinnamon Sugar.  Air fry at 350°F (176°C) for 10
minutes.  Serve and enjoy.  Nutrition: Calories 282 Fat 9g
Carbohydrates 46g Protein 5g

## 101. Air Fried Banana and Walnuts Muffins

Preparation Time: 10 minutes  Cooking Time: 10 minutes
Servings: 2

### Ingredients:

¼ cup flour  ½ tsp. baking powder  ¼ cup mashed banana
¼ cup butter  1 tbsp. chopped walnuts  ¼ cup oats

### Directions:

Spray four muffin molds with cooking spray and set aside.  In a
bowl, mix together mashed bananas, walnuts, sugar, and
butter.  In another bowl, mix oat flour, and baking
powder.  Combine the flour mixture with the banana
mixture.  Pour batter into the prepared muffin mold.  Place in
the air fryer basket and cook at 320°F (160°C) for 10
minutes.  Remove muffins from the air fryer and allow cooling
completely.  Serve and enjoy. Nutrition: Calories 192 Fat 12.3g
Carbohydrates 19.4g Protein 1.9g

## 102. Nutty Mix

Preparation Time: 5 minutes  Cooking Time: 4 minutes
Servings: 6

### Ingredients:

2 cup mix nuts  1 tsp. ground cumin  1 tsp. chili powder  1 tbsp.
melted butter  1 tsp. salt  1 tsp. pepper

## Directions:

Set all ingredients in a large bowl and toss until well coated. Preheat the air fryer at 350°F for 5 minutes. Add mix nuts in the air fryer basket and air fry for 4 minutes. Shake basket halfway through. Serve and enjoy. Nutrition: Calories 316 Fat 29g Carbohydrates 11.3g Protein 7.6g

---

## 103. Vanilla Spiced Soufflé

Preparation Time: 20 minutes  Cooking Time: 32 minutes Servings: 6

### Ingredients:

¼ cup all-purpose flour   1 cup whole milk   2 tsp. Vanilla extract   1 tsp. cream of tartar   1 vanilla bean   4 egg yolks   1-oz. sugar   ¼ cup softened butter   ¼ cup sugar   5 egg whites

### Directions:

Combine flour and butter in a bowl until the mixture becomes a smooth paste.   Set the pan over medium flame to heat the milk. Add sugar and stir until dissolved.   Mix in the vanilla bean and bring to a boil.   Beat the mixture using a wire whisk as you add the butter and flour mixture.   Lower the heat to simmer until thick. Discard the vanilla bean. Turn off the heat.   Place them on an ice bath and allow cooling for 10 minutes.   Grease 6 ramekins with butter. Sprinkle each with a bit of sugar.   Beat the egg yolks in a bowl. Add the vanilla extract and milk mixture. Mix until combined. Whisk together the tartar cream, egg whites, and sugar until it forms medium-stiff peaks. Gradually fold egg whites into the soufflé base. Transfer the mixture to the ramekins. Put 3 ramekins in the cooking basket at a time. Cook for 16 minutes at 330°F. Move to a wire rack for cooling and cook the rest. Sprinkle powdered sugar on top and drizzle with chocolate sauce before serving. Nutrition: Calories 215 Fat 12.2g Carbohydrates 18.98g Protein 6.66g

---

## 104. Chocolate Cup Cakes

Preparation Time: 5 minutes  Cooking Time: 12 minutes
Servings: 6

### Ingredients:

3 eggs   ¼ cup caster sugar   ¼ cup cocoa powder   1 tsp. baking powder   1 cup milk   ¼ tsp. vanilla essence   2 cup all-purpose flour   4 tbsp. Butter

### Directions:

Preheat your Air Fryer to a temperature of 400°F (200°C). Beat eggs with sugar in a bowl until creamy. Add butter and beat again for 1-2 minutes. Now add flour, cocoa powder, milk, and baking powder, and vanilla essence, mix with a spatula. Fill ¾ of muffin tins with the mixture and place them into an Air Fryer basket. Let cook for 12 minutes.  Serve!  Nutrition: Calories 289 Fat 11.5g Carbohydrates 38.94g Protein 8.72g

---

## 105.  Air Baked Cheesecake

Preparation Time: 20 minutes  Cooking Time: 20 minutes Servings: 8-12

### Ingredients:

Crust: ½ cup dates, chopped, soaked in water for at least 15 min., soaking liquid reserved   ½ cup walnuts   1 cup quick oats   Filling: ½ cup vanilla almond milk   ¼ cup coconut palm sugar   ½ cup coconut flour   1 cup cashews, soaked in water for at least 2 hours   1 tsp. vanilla extract   2 tbsp. lemon juice   1 to 2 tsp. grated lemon zest   ½ cup fresh berries or 6 figs, sliced   1 tbsp. arrowroot powder

### Directions:

Make the crust: in a food processor, process together with all the crust ingredients until smooth and press the mixture into the bottom of a spring form pan.   Make the filling: add cashews along with soaking liquid to a blender and process until very smooth; add milk, palm sugar, coconut flour, lemon juice, lemon zest, and vanilla and blend until well combined; add arrowroot and continue blending until mixed and pour into the crust. Smooth the top and cover the spring form pan with foil.   Place the pan in your air fry toaster oven and bake at

375°F for 20 minutes.  Carefully remove the pan from the fryer and remove the foil; let the cake cool completely and top with fruit to serve.  Nutrition: Calories 423 Fat 3.1g Carbohydrates 33.5g Protein 1.2g

## 106.  Air Roasted Nuts

Preparation Time: 10 minutes  Cooking Time: 20 minutes Servings: 8

### Ingredients:

1 cup raw peanuts  ½ tsp. cayenne pepper  3 tsp. seafood seasoning  2 tbsp. olive oil  Salt

### Directions:

Preheat your air fryer toast oven to 320°F.  In a bowl, whisk together cayenne pepper, olive oil, and seafood seasoning stir in peanuts until well coated.   Transfer to the fryer basket and air roast for 10 minutes; toss well and then cook for another 10 minutes.  Transfer the peanuts to a dish and season with salt. Let cool before serving.   Nutrition:  Calories 193 Fat 17.4g Carbohydrates 4.9g Protein 7.4g

## 107. Air Fried White Corn

Preparation Time: 10 minutes  Cooking Time: 40 minutes
Servings: 8

### Ingredients:

2 cups giant white corn    3 tbsp. olive oil   1-½ tsp. sea salt

### Directions:

Soak the corn in a bowl of water for at least 8 hours or overnight; drain and spread in a single layer on a baking tray; pat dry with paper towels.   Preheat your air fryer toast oven to 400°F.   In a bowl, mix corn, olive oil and salt and toss to coat well.   Air fry corn in batches in the preheated air fryer toast oven for 20 minutes, shaking the basket halfway through cooking.   Let the corn cool for at least 20 minutes or until crisp.   Nutrition:  Calories 225 Fat 7.4g Carbohydrates 35.8g Protein 5.9g

## 108. Fruit Cake

Preparation Time: 5 minutes  Cooking Time: 45 minutes
Servings: 4-6

### Ingredients:

Dry Ingredients: ⅛ tsp. sea salt   ½ tsp. baking powder   ½ tsp. baking soda   ½ tsp. ground cardamom   1-¼ cup whole wheat flour   Wet Ingredients: 2 tbsp. coconut oil   ½ cup

unsweetened nondairy milk   2 tbsp. ground flax seeds   ¼ cup
agave   1-½ cups water   Mix-Ins: ½ cup chopped
cranberries   1 cup chopped pear

## Directions:

Grease a Bundt pan; set aside.   In a mixing, mix all dry
ingredients together. In another bowl, combine together the wet
ingredients; whisk the wet ingredients into the dry until
smooth.   Fold in the add-ins and spread the mixture into the
pan; cover with foil.   Place pan in your air fryer toast oven and
add water in the bottom and bake at 370°F for 35
minutes.   When done, use a toothpick to check for doneness. If
it comes out clean, then the cake is ready, if not, bake for 5-10
more minutes, checking frequently to avoid burning.   Remove
the cake and let stand for 10 minutes before transferring from
the pan.   Enjoy!   Nutrition:  Calories 309 Fat 27g
Carbohydrates 14.7g Protein 22.6g